THE
Back
Bible

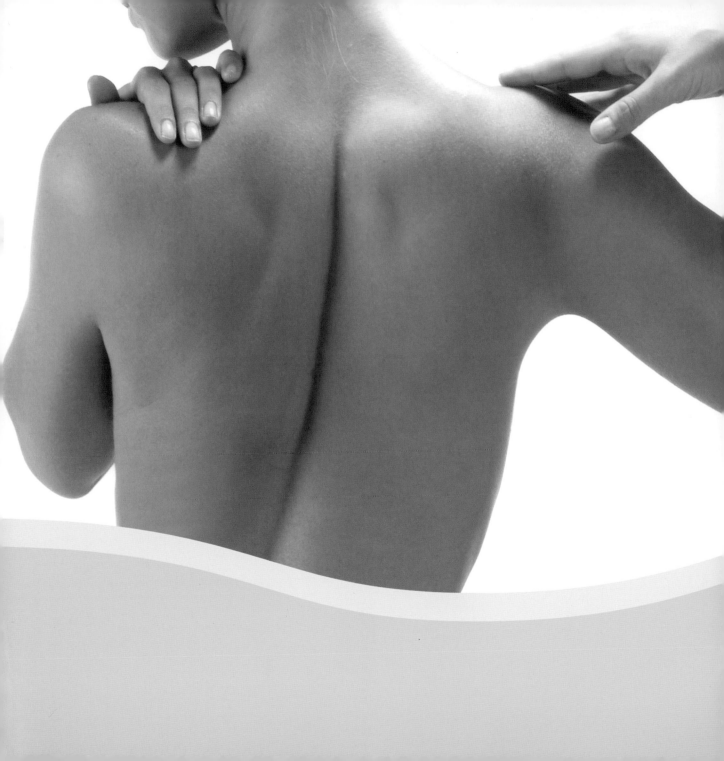

THE
Back
Bible

Dr. Jenny Sutcliffe

Consultants
Daniel E. Gelb, M.D.
Dr. Sarah Jarvis

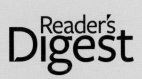

The Reader's Digest Association, Inc.
New York, NY/Montreal/Sydney/Mumbai

Conceived, edited, and designed by
Marshall Editions
The Old Brewery
6 Blundell Street
London N7 9BH
www.marshalleditions.com

Publisher James Ashton-Tyler
Editorial Director Sorrel Wood
Project Editor Cathy Meeus
Copy Editor Nigel Perryman
Art Direction Schermuly Design Co.
Photography Simon Pask

Front cover images: iStock
Back cover images: Shutterstock or as credited on page 224

A READER'S DIGEST BOOK

Reader's Digest is a registered trademark of The Reader's Digest Association, Inc.

FOR READER'S DIGEST
Project Editor Ellen Michaud
Manager, English Book Editorial, Reader's Digest Canada Pamela Johnson
Project Designer Jennifer Tokarski
Senior Art Director George McKeon
Associate Publisher, Trade Publishing Rosanne McManus
President and Publisher, Trade Publishing Harold Clarke

ISBN 978-1-60652-254-7 (hardcover)
ISBN 978-1-60652-509-8 (paperback)

We are committed to both the quality of our products and the service we provide to our customers. We value your comments, so please feel free to contact us.

The Reader's Digest Association, Inc.
Adult Trade Publishing
44 South Broadway
White Plains, NY 10601

For more Reader's Digest products and information, visit our website:
www.rd.com (in the United States)
www.readersdigest.ca (in Canada)
www.readersdigest.co.uk (in the UK)
www.readersdigest.com.au (in Australia)
www.readersdigest.co.nz (in New Zealand)
www.rdasia.com (in Asia)

Originated in Hong Kong by Modern Age Repro House Ltd.
Printed and bound in China by 1010 Printing International Ltd.

1 3 5 7 9 10 8 6 4 2

NOTE TO OUR READERS
The information in this book should not be substituted for, or used to alter, medical therapy without your doctor's advice. For a specific health problem, consult your physician for guidance. Please consult your doctor before attempting any of the exercises featured in this book.

Contents

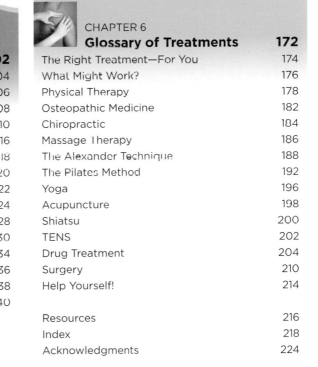

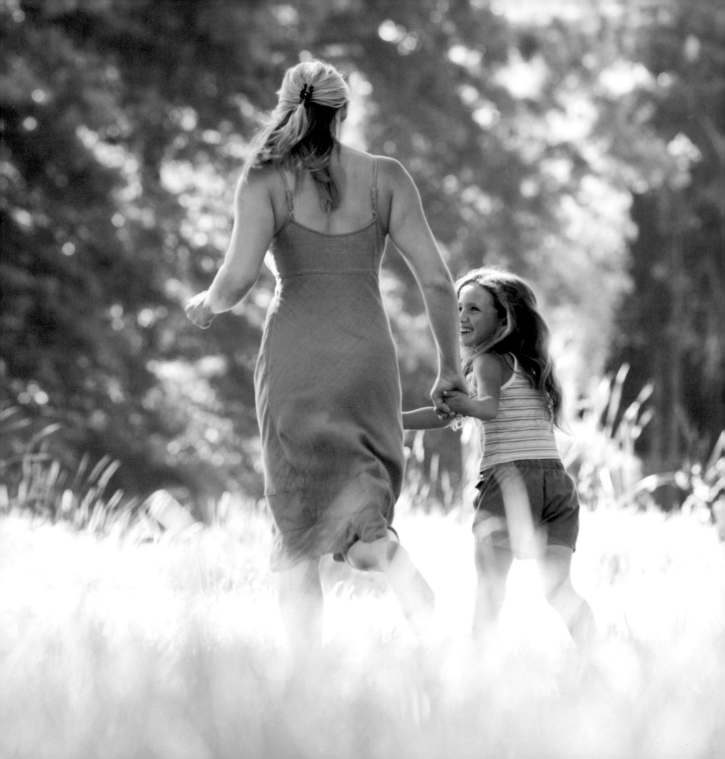

Introduction

Ever had a bad back? Nearly everybody has. In fact, Americans spend an astounding $86 billion a year on dealing with their backs—trying to stop them from interfering with work, leisure, and just normal day-to-day life.

The causes of back problems are primarily bad posture and activity-related mishaps. If you haven't moved a muscle for months, for example, walking around with slouched shoulders then suddenly becoming a weekend gardener and digging up your yard can trash your back.

But from minor strains to more serious trouble, there's usually no need to worry. Most back problems resolve in a few days, and if they don't there's a whole range of treatments that will help clear them up in no time. While it's always wise to check out any back pain with your doctor, this book will share with you what you can do to help yourself, how a range of treatments work, and how to choose from among them.

Occasionally, things can be more serious. Muscles, joints, ligaments, and tendons can all be challenged by incorrect patterns of movement, and bad posture or disease can play a part in disrupting your back's normal function. Even so, there are treatments your doctor or physical therapist can recommend that will have you walking tall in no time.

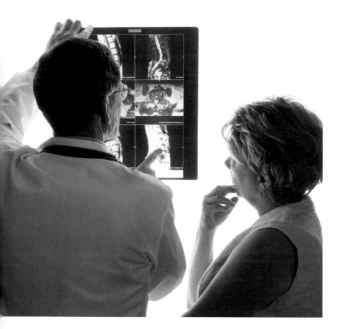

Getting the most from this book *The Back Bible* is designed to be your guide to maintaining optimum back health. It tells you how your back works, what can go wrong with it, what to do when a problem arises, and what your options are. But, above all, the emphasis is on prevention: how you can tailor your life and your environment at work and at home to minimize the possibility of hurting your back. From essential advice on posture to detailed information about how to care for your back while sitting at a desk, traveling in a car, gardening, or lifting and carrying, this book will help keep your back in shape.

Understanding the fundamentals In Chapter 1, *Back to Basics*, you'll find a wealth of information on the structure and healthy functioning of your back to help you understand how this impressive piece of engineering works. There's also an overview of the kinds of things that can go wrong with your back.

What's my problem? Diagnosis of back problems is the job of your physician, but in *How Do I Know What's Wrong?* (page 38) you'll find helpful advice on distinguishing problems that require immediate or even emergency medical attention from those that simply require timely advice from your family physician. What's more, you'll discover how a diagnosis is made and the tests that may be required in *An Expert Assessment* (page 42).

If you want to know more about the anatomy or the conditions that affect specific areas of the spine, you'll find the information you seek in Chapters 3 and 4 (*Neck and Shoulders; Middle and Lower Back*). Each of these chapters contains an introduction to the anatomical structures in these areas, followed by sections that describe the conditions that affect each region of the spine. And there are exercise tips to keep it in great shape.

It could occur anywhere There are a number of conditions that either affect the whole back or make their presence felt anywhere along the spine. Chapter 2, *The Whole Back*, is the place to find information on these disorders.

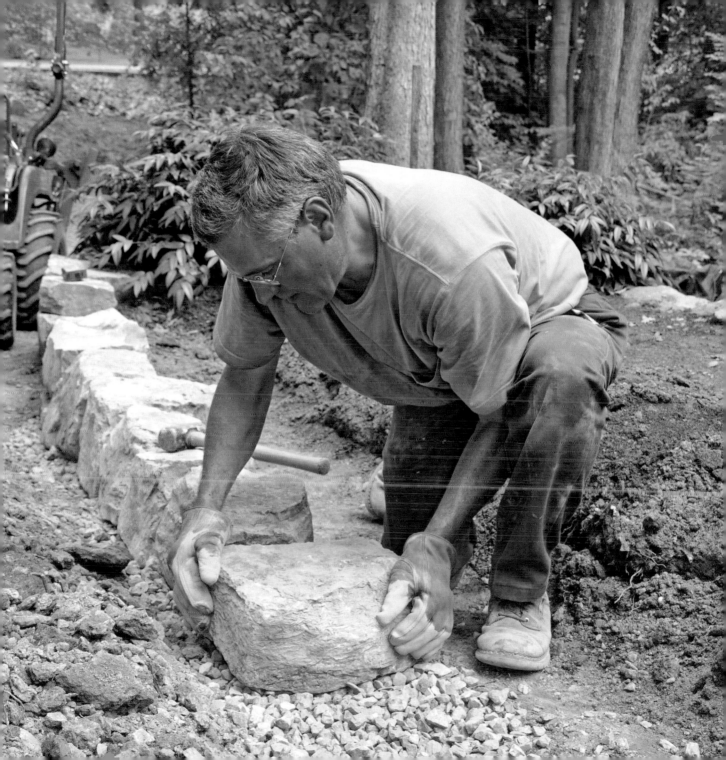

Avoiding trouble Of course, prevention is better than cure. In Chapter 5, *The Healthy Back*, you'll find practical tips to maintain a strong, supple, flexible back both at home and at work—including information on nutrients that may support back health.

Healthy moves This entire book is packed with effective exercises illustrated with step-by-step photographs to help you maintain back health and alleviate aches and pains. Exercises that are designed to address specific problems are carefully detailed by a physical therapist, while exercises for maintaining back strength and mobility can be found in Chapter 5, *The Healthy Back* (page 164).

What's the treatment? Once your physician has diagnosed a back problem, the next stage is to decide on a treatment. Your physician will advise you, but to help you make your choice, Chapter 6, *Glossary of Treatments*, outlines the principles behind many and explains how they work. From physical therapy and medication to Pilates and shiatsu, your questions will be answered.

Use Common Sense ▸▸

The exercises in this book have been recommended by physical therapists for general back health or for the relief of the conditions specified. But before you exercise be sure to take note of these commonsense guidelines:

■ Consult your physician before trying any exercise if you have a pre-existing back condition or other health problem.

■ Warm up before starting any exercise (follow the routine on page 96) and relax (as described on page 162) for five minutes afterward. Make sure that your room is warm in order to help your muscles stretch and relax, and adequately aired, so that you are able to take in sufficient oxygen to maximize muscle efficiency.

■ Stop if the pain starts to become worse during exercise and seek the advice of your physician.

■ Don't push through any pain: the stretches should be smooth and not jerky. Continue through your full range of movement but no further—any more and you risk triggering the "muscle stretch reflex," which causes an overstretched muscle to contract further.

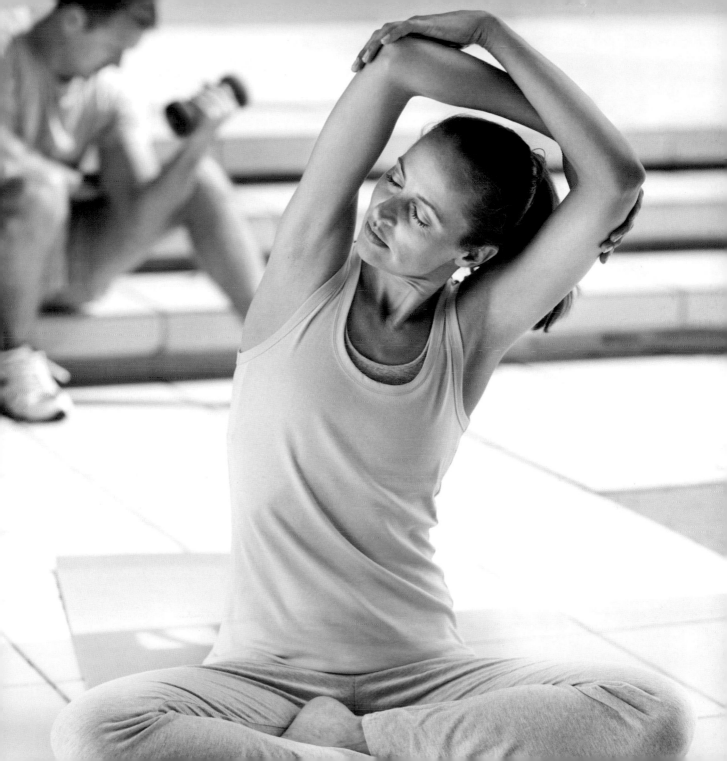

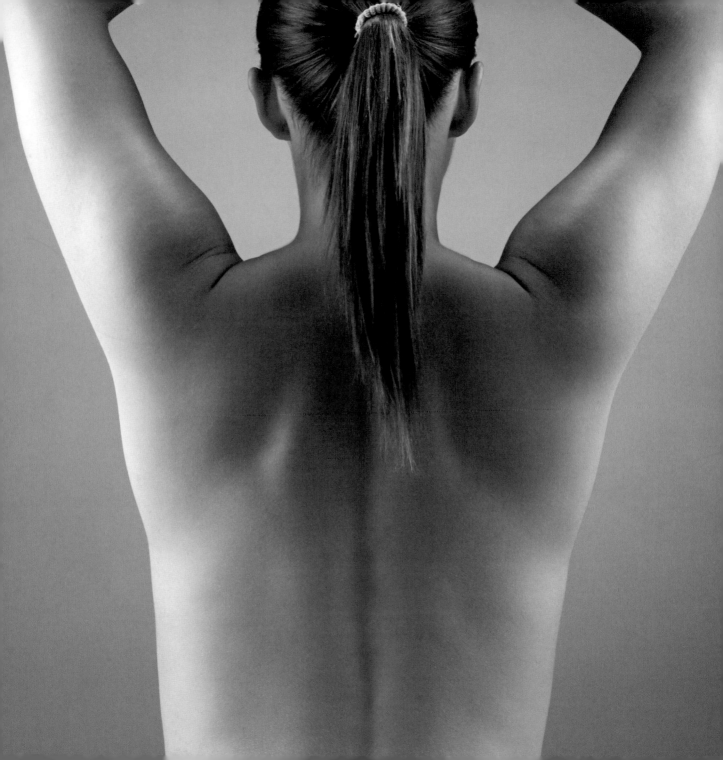

Chapter 1

Back to Basics

The segmented structure of the back and its complex system of joints provide the strength and flexibility we need in our daily lives. In this chapter you'll find a full description of the anatomy of the back, including bones, joints, muscles, and ligaments, as well as the spinal cord and nerves. You'll also learn how the back works and how it sometimes can be damaged by injury and disease. Last but not least, there's information on the causes of back problems and what to do if you're affected.

The Living Back

The human back has both the flexibility we need to perform complex and precise movements and sufficient strength to anchor our limbs and enable us to stand upright. Even so, many of us suffer from back pain, which is usually the result of misuse or neglect owing to our busy lifestyles.

Of all the elements that comprise our backs, the spine is the most elegant in term of its design. It consists of 33 individual bones called vertebrae.

Elements of flexibilty As a whole, the spine allows sufficient flexibility to make twisting and bending possible, even though the movement permitted between individual vertebrae is often small. In fact, the sacral vertebrae and some of the coccygeal ones allow no movement at all. The movement of the spine also allows the ribs to rise and fall when we breathe in and out. But the flexibility does not come at the expense of strength: the spine is still strong enough to support the head and anchor the muscles that move the lower limbs. It also contains and protects the spinal cord, which carries the nerves that connect the brain to the nerves that serve the rest of the body.

The most numerous of the vertebrae are those from the base of the neck to the middle of the chest: the thoracic vertebrae. Each one is separated from the vertebrae above and below it by an intervertebral disk of cartilage that makes up about a quarter of the spine's length; the disks act both as shock absorbers and ball bearings, allowing the spine to twist and bend.

THE SPINE
There are five groups of vertebrae: cervical, in the neck; thoracic, in the chest; lumbar, in the lower back; sacral, between the buttocks; and the coccyx (tailbone).

A VERTEBRA
A vertebra of the thoracic spine is illustrated below. The body of thc vertebra faces inward toward the abdominal cavity and the processes face outward.

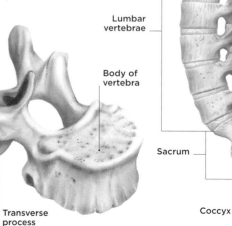

Cervical vertebrae

Thoracic vertebrae

Lumbar vertebrae

Body of vertebra

Sacrum

Coccyx

Spinous process

Transverse process

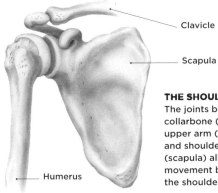

Clavicle

Scapula

Humerus

THE SHOULDER
The joints between the collarbone (clavicle), upper arm (humerus), and shoulder blade (scapula) allow movement but give the shoulder strength.

Each vertebra also has a number of joints—not just the intervertebral ones, but synovial joints (that is, lubricated by synovial fluid, which, rather like a car's engine oil, helps to reduce wear and tear when bone moves against bone). The most important are the facet joints (page 16). The terms "facet joints" and "Z-joints," as they are also known, are shorthand for their proper anatomical name of "zygapophysial joints." They are bony catches that prevent each vertebra from slipping off the next one, making the spine into a bony chain that, again, is flexible yet strong.

Taller in the Morning! ➤

The center of the cartilaginous disks between the vertebrae is classically likened to the chewy center of a hard candy, and is 85 percent water. During the day our upright stance means that the weight of the bones in the spinal column compresses each disk by as much as 10 percent. But during sleep the pressure is reduced and the disks reabsorb water, with the result that you can wake up as much as an inch taller than when you went to bed.

Shouldering the strain It may seem strange to talk about the shoulder in a book about the back, but the two are not only linked anatomically but through their working relationship. This means that many problems in the spine can make themselves felt in the shoulder and vice versa. The shoulder joint (see left and page 88) comprises the associated back bones, the collarbone (clavicle) and the shoulder blade (scapula), and the upper arm bone (humerus). Most of the muscles that anchor the joint originate in the back and, in particular, in the scapula. Therefore the joint's performance and the movements of the arm are inextricably linked with those of the back.

A protective basin While the back and shoulders anchor the arms, the pelvis anchors the legs. In Latin, pelvis means "basin," which is a fitting term for the protective housing of so many vital organs. But it can also be thought of as part of the lower back, not just because its upper rim is part of the back, but because of the strength and stability it provides as the anchoring point for the legs. These are joined to the pelvis at the hip sockets.

THE PELVIS
The pelvis anchors the legs to the spine.

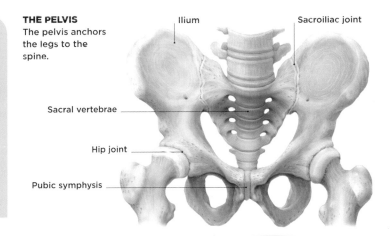

Ilium

Sacroiliac joint

Sacral vertebrae

Hip joint

Pubic symphysis

Flexible and Stable

The individual bones of the spine—the vertebrae—are linked by a complex system of joints that provide the flexibility we need to twist and turn without killing our backs. Yet the spine also provides the stability required to fulfill its role as an anchoring structure for our arms and legs.

Fitting together Along with the specialized structures of the bony vertebrae, the spinal joints are formed by soft tissues, mainly cartilage and ligaments. In a healthy back, each vertebra is separated from its neighbor by a cushioning pad of cartilaginous material, known as an intervertebral disk. The three bony projections from the back of the body of the vertebrae, known as the processes (see page 14), are also joined. Ligaments provide a firm but somewhat flexible link between the processes of adjoining vertebrae, as well as along the length of the spine.

Disks Each intervertebral disk has a soft gel-like interior (nucleus pulposus) enclosed within a tough outer layer (anular fibrosus). It allows for movement by molding itself to the space available as the vertebrae move in relation to each other, preventing direct contact—and therefore wear—between the bony surfaces. The disks depend on rest and movement to help them maintain their sponginess. Rest also enables the disks to recover their shape following periods of pressure on the spine from everyday activities. When disks lose fluid-content, a natural consequence of aging, they cease to protect

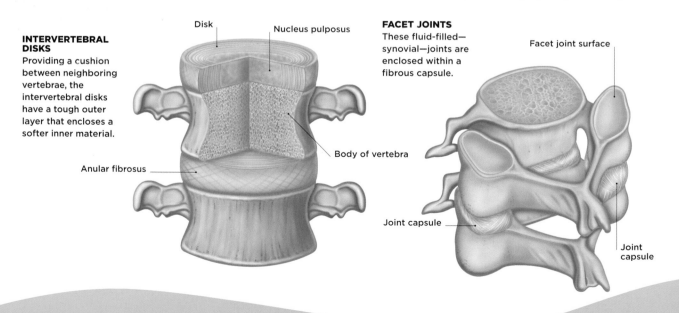

INTERVERTEBRAL DISKS
Providing a cushion between neighboring vertebrae, the intervertebral disks have a tough outer layer that encloses a softer inner material.

Disk

Nucleus pulposus

Anular fibrosus

Body of vertebra

FACET JOINTS
These fluid-filled—synovial—joints are enclosed within a fibrous capsule.

Facet joint surface

Joint capsule

Joint capsule

the joint as effectively, and bone changes leading to increasing stiffness, and, over time, fusion of the vertebrae, can result. If they are overstressed they can also protrude from the joint margins (prolapse) and may cause pressure on nearby nerves. (See also *Pressure on the Nerve Roots*, page 116.)

Facet joints Also known as Z-joints, these are tiny joints between the transverse processes on the backs of adjoining vertebrae (see page 14). They both permit and limit forward bending and backward flexion of the spine.

There are four facet surfaces on each vertebra and the surface of each is protected by a layer of cartilage. A fluid-filled fibrous capsule encloses each facet joint. The fluid provides friction-reducing lubrication to assist smooth movement and prevent wear. Joints that are lubricated by fluid in this way are known as synovial joints. Wear on the facet joints or inflammation resulting from rheumatoid arthritis (page 62) is a common cause of back pain.

Ligaments These are bands of strong, fibrous tissue that run between the bones to reinforce and protect joints from excessive movement. Longitudinal ligaments run lengthways from top to bottom of the spine along the front, back, and sides of the vertebral bodies and shorter ligaments connect the processes and facet joints.

Ligaments are slightly elastic. They allow movement but only within a safe range. When you bend forward, the ligaments stretch until they are taut. Once tight, they prevent any further movement at the joint. If they didn't, other soft tissues, such as your muscles and disks, would have to hold your vertebrae together—something they're not constructed to do.

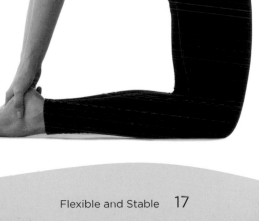

BEND AND STRETCH
The spine permits a surprising range of movement, but most of us lose this flexibility unless we regularly practice yoga or similar forms of exercise.

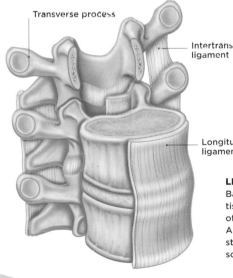

Transverse process

Intertransverse ligament

Longitudinal ligament

LINES OF LIGAMENTS
Bands of tough, fibrous tissue bind the elements of the spine together. A limited amount of stretchiness allows some flexibility.

Muscle Up

Movement of the back is generated by the muscles that surround the spine and abdomen. These fibrous tissues also give support and strength to the entire structure. Arranged in symmetrical pairs on each side of the spine, the muscles of the back criss-cross the trunk from the shoulder and pelvis to the spine and ribs. No muscle crosses the midline of the spine.

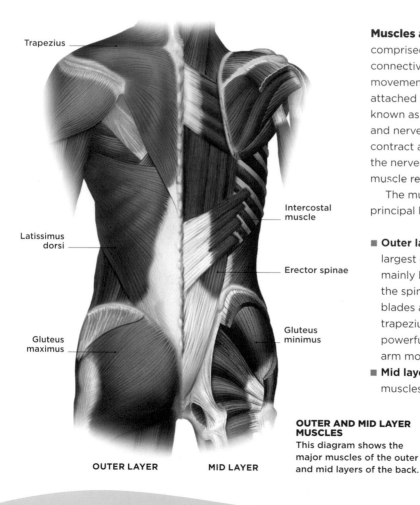

Trapezius

Latissimus dorsi

Gluteus maximus

Intercostal muscle

Erector spinae

Gluteus minimus

OUTER LAYER　　　**MID LAYER**

OUTER AND MID LAYER MUSCLES
This diagram shows the major muscles of the outer and mid layers of the back.

Muscles and tendons Individual muscles are comprised of bundles of long, thin fibers bound by connective tissue. The muscles that control back movement are skeletal muscles—that is, they are attached at each end to a bone by fibrous cords known as tendons. With their rich supply of blood and nerves, the muscle fibers are designed to contract and relax according to the prompting by the nerves. When a muscle contracts, the opposing muscle relaxes, and the bone or joint moves.

The muscles of the back are arranged in three principal layers:

- **Outer layer** The muscles in this layer are the largest of those that control the back. They are mainly broad, triangular sheets of muscle that join the spinal processes (see page 14) to the shoulder blades and shoulder joint. They include the trapezius and the latissimus dorsi ("lats"). These powerful muscles keep the trunk stable during arm movements.
- **Mid layer** These are mainly strap-shaped muscles, such as the erector spinae, that fan out from the pelvis and attach to the vertebrae, ribs, and skull.
- **Deep layer** The deepest muscles are also the shortest. Muscles in this layer run between the vertebrae

and maintain the alignment of the spine. Importantly, they contract to stabilize the spine before movement.

Don't forget your stomach The muscles of the abdomen are essential partners to those of the back. They exert a counteracting force to the forward and backward pull of the back muscles. Contraction of the abdominal muscles pulls the ribcage closer to the pelvis, which allows the spine to bend forward. The abdominals also work in conjunction with the back muscles to produce twisting movements.

Contraction of the large abdominal muscles increases the pressure within the abdominal cavity, which provides additional support for the spine. This can be critical for sharing the strain when the spine is under stress—say, when lifting a heavy load.

Gird your loins One deep muscle that is of particular importance for the back is the psoas, or loin muscle. This long, thick abdominal muscle runs from the lumbar vertebrae, inside the pelvis, to the top of the femur, below the hip joint (in combination with the iliacus muscle, it makes up the illiopsoas muscle). It flexes the hips and thighs and helps control lower back posture. When it contracts, it compresses the disks between the lumbar vertebrae. Those who spend many hours a day sitting, often suffer from shortened iliopsoas muscles, which can contribute to poor posture. (See also *Take the Right Posture*, page 148.)

Know your fascia The fascia is a thin film of connective tissue that envelops and separates everything in your body from head to foot. Each muscle, and every muscle fiber within it, has a fascial surround, so that the two are functionally

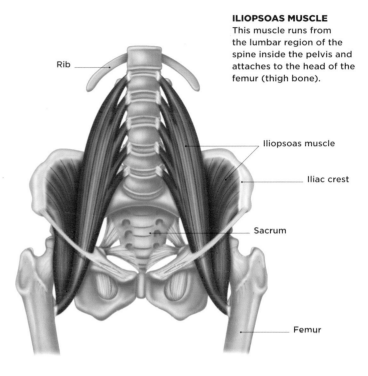

ILIOPSOAS MUSCLE
This muscle runs from the lumbar region of the spine inside the pelvis and attaches to the head of the femur (thigh bone).

Rib

Iliopsoas muscle

Iliac crest

Sacrum

Femur

bound together. Check out a cooked chicken leg: if you carefully pull it apart, you'll see the fascia—a thin layer of tissue separating the different muscles.

The fascia itself is made up of lots of thin layers of wriggly collagen fibers. When a muscle lengthens, the collagen fibers stretch out until they are straight, after which they resist further movement. Normal, healthy fascia stretches and contracts and allows muscles and other structures to glide smoothly over each other. But when it is static or connected to a tight muscle, fascia tends to lose its elasticity and thickens, and fascia that is overstretched can tear more easily. This results in pain and inflammation.

Channels of Communication

The bony structure of the spine does more than hold your skeleton together. It also provides a vital protective channel for the spinal cord—the communications superhighway between the brain and the rest of your body.

The importance of the spinal cord cannot be overemphasized. A key part of the central nervous system that also includes the brain, it is the route by which all signals from the brain travel to the rest of the body and through which sensory signals from the peripheral nervous system travel back to the brain. The complex shape of the vertebrae creates a central channel in the spine within its bony framework. Additional openings on each side of the spine between the vertebrae provide access points for the spinal nerves to emerge along the length of the cord.

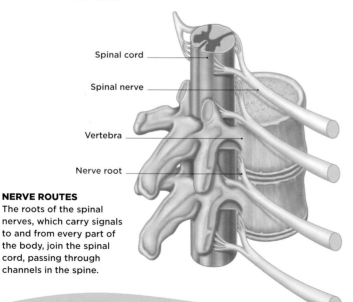

Spinal cord

Spinal nerve

Vertebra

Nerve root

NERVE ROUTES
The roots of the spinal nerves, which carry signals to and from every part of the body, join the spinal cord, passing through channels in the spine.

Structure of the spinal cord The spinal cord is cylindrical in shape. It's composed of an inner core of nerve fibers surrounded by blood vessels and enclosed within a three-layered casing containing cerebrospinal fluid—the same fluid that surrounds the brain. This forms an additional protective layer.

The spinal nerves Emerging at intervals from the spinal cord, these are the conduit for nerve signals to and from specific regions of the body (see right). Broadly speaking, those emerging from the neck and shoulder region of the spine serve the head, neck, and arms; those emerging from the thoracic region serve the trunk; and those in the lumbar region serve the area around the waist and legs. The spinal cord ends near the top of the lumbar spine. Below this is a branching structure, the cauda equina (horse tail), which serves the legs, buttocks, and lower abdomen. Neurologists can pinpoint the location of a damaged spinal nerve from the location of any symptoms being felt.

Types of nerve fiber There are two different types of nerve fiber, each of which is responsible for relaying a different type of signal.

- **Motor nerves** Sometimes known as efferent nerves, these carry signals from the brain that trigger the contraction of muscles to produce movement. These voluntary muscles are under conscious control, in contrast to the involuntary muscles over which we have no control, such as those of the heart or digestive system. The latter are controlled by a separate nervous system, known as the autonomic nervous system.

■ **Sensory nerves** Sometimes known as afferent nerves, these send messages from the sensory nerve endings in the body to the brain, where they are interpreted so that they can be consciously understood. A sensation-producing stimulus may occur, for example, in the hand, but it is "felt" in the brain.

The spinal nerves are comprised of both motor and sensory fibers.

Cervical nerves

Thoracic nerves

Lumbar nerves

Sacral and cocygeal nerves

Cauda equina

AREAS OF CONTROL
The color coding on the diagram of the spine (left) and the illustrations (below) indicates the areas of the body controlled by the nerves that emerge from each region of the spine: Mauve—controlled by the cervical nerves. Purple—controlled by the thoracic nerves. Blue—controlled by the cauda equina emerging from the lumbar region. Green—controlled by the cauda equina emerging from the sacrum (tailbone).

Brain

Cauda equina

Spinal cord

Sciatic nerve

CAUDA EQUINA
This branching nerve structure starts at the base of the spinal cord in the lumbar region. It includes the nerves that serve the legs.

Back in Action

To understand how the back works as a unit, we need to look at the mechanical forces that affect it as we live our daily lives—and to appreciate how the human back has evolved over the millennia to cope with them. The science that this involves is known as "biomechanics."

In relation to the back, biomechanics is the study of how gravity, the action of muscles, and life events affect the bones, joints, muscles, and ligaments of which it is comprised. An understanding of biomechanics is important because the cause of a

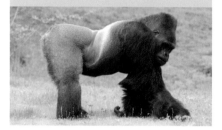

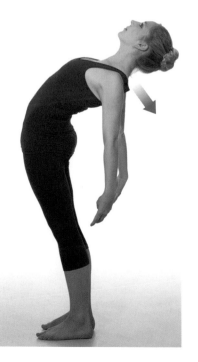

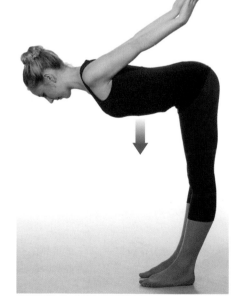

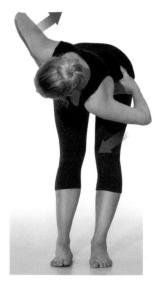

back problem is more often than not a disruption of the normal biomechanical system as a result of genetics, disease, aging, and the way we move.

The forces at play A "force" is something that puts pressure on a structure and there is one obvious force that affects the back throughout life—gravity, which compresses the vertebrae and the intervertebral disks. Compression is a problem unique to humans, who, unlike our cousins the apes, always walk upright. Unfortunately, our backs have had to evolve with some degree of compromise to make this possible, because a structure that provided enough rigidity to counteract the pressure of gravity would reduce the flexibility we need to perform the movements required in our daily lives.

RANGE OF MOVEMENT
The spine permits a varied range of movement: forward, backward, rotation, and sideways.

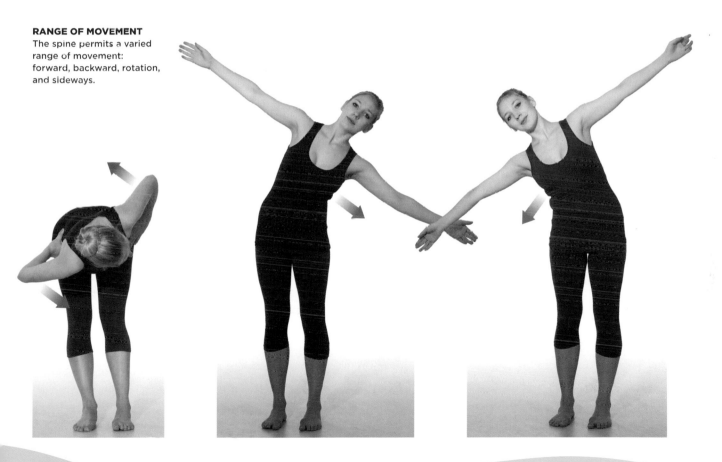

The diagrams (right) illustrate the effects of the forces to which our spines are subject as we go about our daily activities. The neutral position, in which no forces are present, is shown for comparison.

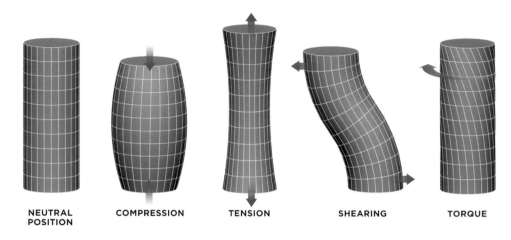

NEUTRAL POSITION **COMPRESSION** **TENSION** **SHEARING** **TORQUE**

Partly as a result of our upright posture, our backs have had to cope with other forces as well as compression: tension, shear, and torque.

- **Tension** This is a stretching force applied to the spine, often by the force of gravity—for example, if you hang from a bar in a gym.
- **Shearing forces** These are exerted when you lean to one side or the other and try to force the spine out of its normal perpendicular axis.
- **Torque** This force tries to rotate the components of the spine around their usual axis.

To resist these forces the spine has developed a number of defensive mechanisms. Without them, vertebrae would be moved out of alignment, ligaments would tear, and disks would be damaged. But these defenses can be broken down by the strength of the forces involved or may degenerate to the extent that damage is possible.

Columns of control The spine functions as two "columns" (anterior/front and posterior/back) in a way that maximizes strength and flexibility

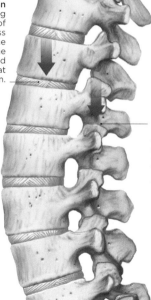

Front column
Forces acting on the front of the spine pass through the bodies of the vertebrae and the disks that separate them.

Rear column
Forces acting on the rear of the spine pass through the facet joints that link the spinal processes.

DUAL CONTROLS
The forces on the back are moderated by the twin structures: the vertebral bodies and disks (front) and the jointed spinal processes (back).

and guards against these forces. The front, load-bearing structure comprises the vertebrae and their intervertebral disks, while the back structure, often called a "tension band," is made up of the spinal processes, facet joints, and ligaments. (For more information on these structures, see pages 12–16.)

Balancing the load Our daily activities put pressure on the spine's supporting structures, but they are designed to withstand them. Problems arise, however, when the structures are distorted by poor posture (page 148), conditions like osteoarthritis that cause their degeneration, or are not protected by us as we move through life lifting this, balancing that, and twisting through it all.

The neutral zone Fortunately, a number of research studies have shown that "neutral zone" (NZ) exercises can help build your capacity to withstand stresses on the back and so prevent low-back injuries and pain. These are exercises in which you limit the range of spinal motion so there are no significant stresses on the spinal ligaments or disks. You can limit these stresses by trying to maintain the normal lumbar curve in the lower spine and pelvis during any movement. Think about it this

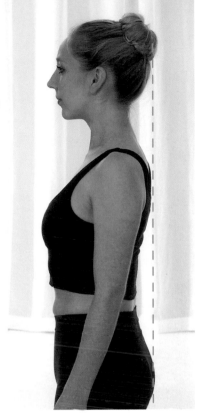

NEUTRAL POSITION
In the neutral position, the natural curves of the spine provide optimum protection for the back against stress and strain.

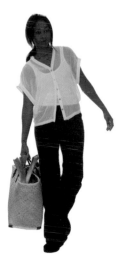

DAILY STRESS
Even a simple activity like carrying a shopping bag can exert damaging stress on the spine.

way: if you flex your lumbar spine, you put your ligaments, disks, and muscles under pressure, and put the muscles that extend the spine in the lower back at a mechanical disadvantage. They cannot help reduce shear forces, so the spine is more likely to be injured. When in a neutral position, the pelvis can tilt in equal amounts of flexion, with the bottom tucked under, or extension—the "swayback" position. Practicing the lying and sitting pelvic tilt exercises on page 134 will help you achieve this neutral position, and over time will make correct posture second nature, which reduces your risk of injury.

What Can Go Wrong?

Lots. Your back and the problems that may affect it change at each stage of life. As you move through childhood, engage in new activities, have a family, and grow older, you and your back will encounter new challenges. On the following pages you'll find an overview of the causes of the back problems that can occur.

Some back problems can be prevented, but others are the result of an unavoidable accident or illness. Most can affect people of any age and may occur in any area of the back. More detailed descriptions of these conditions as they affect specific areas of the back and suggestions for exercises that may help are given in later chapters.

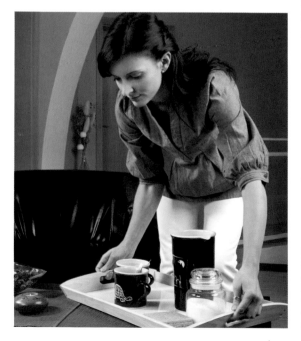

EVERYDAY STRAIN
Sometimes a simple, everyday activity, such as lifting a tray in an awkward way, can leave you with days of back pain from muscle and ligament strain.

Muscle and ligament strain As we have seen, the muscles and ligaments of the back can accommodate a wide variety of movements (see *Flexible and Stable*, page 17), but can be damaged if they are stretched beyond their accustomed range, leading to strains that tear muscle fibers. In response, the affected muscles often go into spasm—becoming painfully stiff—until the damage has healed. The following are leading causes of muscle-related back problems:

- **Strenuous exercise** Especially if you are not accustomed to it and have not warmed up properly beforehand, this is often responsible for minor muscle strains. Sports that involve twisting movements—racquetball or tennis, for example—can also strain muscles and ligaments that are not sufficiently strong or flexible.
- **Lifting incorrectly** This is another key cause of muscle and ligament strain—and it needn't involve hugely heavy loads. Many occupations involve a great deal of lifting and carrying, and over time, this kind of repeated strain can take its toll on your back. For example, wait staff in restaurants, who have

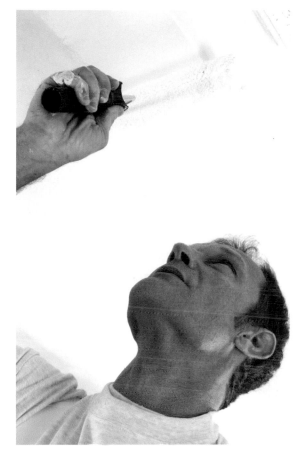

RISK OF REPETITION
Repetitive actions, such as those that are needed for tasks such as house-painting, are a leading cause of muscle strain in the back.

- **Repetitive actions** These involve making the same set of movements for an extended period of time and can lead to muscle stiffness and spasm. This is one of the main causes of back pain related to the workplace. Examples of repetitive actions include activities that you may perform in the course of work or at home, such as house-painting or carpentry, in which you repeatedly make the same movement.
- **Carrying excess weight** Whether as a result of excess body fat or pregnancy (see *If You're Pregnant*, page 130), an increase in weight, especially in the abdominal area, can increase the strain on your back muscles. It can overstretch the abdominal muscles and make them less effective in sharing the work of lifting. (See also *Lighten Up*, page 158.)

Stress-related muscle spasm We all suffer from psychological stress at some time, and some of us lead lives that seem to be filled with events and worries that keep us tense. Unfortunately, it's very common for stress to find physical expression in the form of back, neck, or shoulder pain. Physiologically what happens is that in response to a particular stressor, the "fight or flight" response kicks in. Hormones are released that tighten the muscles—just in case you should have to confront a threat for which a physical response may be appropriate. The result can be pain—sometimes severe. (See also *Be Relaxed*, page 162.)

to twist and turn while carrying trays for long shifts, often suffer from chronic back trouble. If your technique for lifting is faulty, you can easily end up with a seriously painful and stiff back. (For more information about correct lifting technique, see *How to Avoid Strain*, page 152.)

Muscle imbalance A healthy back is a symmetrical back –that is, when viewed from the back, the spine is straight and the muscles that serve it are evenly developed on both sides. This is not always the case. In many of us, poor posture or habitual movements that are necessitated by our work lead

BACK TO SPORT
Exercise is great for your general health, but some sports can put your back at risk if you overwork certain muscles.

to muscular imbalances that create strain on the back. For example, tennis players are likely to have more highly developed muscles on the side on which they habitually hold the racket. Over time the pull exerted by the muscles on the stronger side can strain the opposing muscles on the weaker side. The solution is to embark on a program of exercise to build up muscle strength in the less-developed arm and the trunk on that side. A physical therapist will be able to suggest exercises that will do this.

Accidents and injuries Some of the most common back problems, especially among younger people, are the result of a fall or other accident. A fall can bruise the back and, in more serious cases, the vertebrae can be fractured. The immediate concern with a fractured vertebra is that the spinal cord that it encloses will be damaged, creating a risk of long-term disability. Appropriate action in the case of falls is discussed on page 38.

Whiplash is a type of injury that is frequently caused by car crashes. A sudden jolt causes the spine (usually in the neck region) to jerk back then forward beyond its normal range of movement, stretching and straining the supporting ligaments, muscles, and facet joints. The result is neck and back pain, stiffness, and often headaches. Be aware: whiplash always requires assessment by a physician.

Disk problems Many people are familiar with the term "slipped disk" in the context of disabling back pain. In fact, this term is a misnomer. The condition is more accurately referred to as a prolapsed disk and describes a situation in which a disk between two vertebrae (page 16) protrudes from between the vertebrae and the soft, cushioning material inside can be leaking out. This can put pressure on the spinal cord and nearby nerves, producing pain

and other symptoms. It usually occurs as a result of long-term stress on the back that has caused the inner material of the disks to lose resilience and the outer covering of one or more of the disks to be damaged.

Facet joint damage These tiny joints between neighboring vertebrae (see *Flexible and Stable*, page 16) are a major cause of long-term back pain. The facet joints can be damaged if they are pressed together too tightly. This can occur if:

- The disks between vertebrae shrink, narrowing the gap between the vertebrae.
- The surrounding ligaments become slack, as can happen in older people.
- You sit in one place for an extended time.
- You have poor posture or wear high heels.

Bone degeneration The vertebrae are made of the same material as bones elsewhere in the body and are therefore vulnerable to similar types of bone degeneration. Bone can degenerate as a response to poor diet, little exercise, or simply as part of the aging process. These problems are discussed in the section on osteoporosis (page 68).

Nerve damage Because the spine provides a protective channel for the main nerve pathways of the body, it is not surprising that many problems originating in the bones and soft tissues of the spine can also have an impact on the nearby nerves. For example, inflammation of the tissues around a damaged facet joint can cause pressure on a spinal nerve emerging from that point in the spine. Similarly, a prolapsed disk can put pressure on the spinal cord. And, importantly, spinal injuries can also damage the nerves themselves.

Tell-tale symptoms that a nerve may be affected include numbness and tingling and/or shooting pains. The precise location of the symptoms depends on the area of the back and therefore the nerves affected. Damage to certain nerves can also affect the functioning of various organs. You'll find more information about how nerve damage may show itself in *Cervical Nerve Root Problems* (page 82) and *Pressure on the Nerve Roots* (page 116).

Inflammatory conditions Since the spine is part of the musculoskeletal system, it is subject to the wide range of conditions that can affect the bones, muscles, and joints in other parts of the body. These include those that cause joint inflammation.

Inflammation is usually characterized by swelling, redness, and heat in the affected area. It is the body's normal response to attack by germs or other "foreign" substances. Unfortunately, this response can also occur when there is no threat, or if the body perceives the threat as coming from its own tissues. Inflammatory conditions that occur as a result of this "mistaken" response are known as autoimmune disorders. The main autoimmune disorders that commonly affect the back are rheumatoid arthritis (page 62) and ankylosing spondylitis (page 66).

Repeated damage or trauma to body tissues can also cause inflammation. In the spine, this type of inflammation is most often the result of osteoarthritis, in which the cushioning between the joints degenerates and the joints become inflamed as a result of excessive wear and tear. (For more information on this condition, see page 58.)

Infection Both bacterial and viral infections involving the back are rare, but can be serious as they can affect the spinal cord and, in some cases, the brain. Meningitis is the most significant of these. This infection of the membranes that enclose the brain can sometimes cause neck and back pain and stiffness, as well as a severe headache, fever, vomiting, and/or aversion to bright light. Meningitis can be a medical emergency, so it is important to call your doctor immediately if you experience any of these symptoms.

Infection within the bony canal surrounding the spinal cord, an epidural abscess, can also cause back pain along with fever and extreme tiredness. Less common than meningitis, this condition also demands prompt medical attention.

Pregnancy and back pain Most women experience back pain at some point during the course of their pregnancy. The lower back is the area most commonly affected. The reasons for this are twofold. The impact of the increasing size of a pregnant woman's belly has already been mentioned (see *Carrying excess weight*, page 27). Not only does the added weight in this area affect the muscle tone of the abdomen, but it also alters the mom-to-be's center of gravity and therefore her posture. As a result, muscle strain in the lumbar region is not uncommon.

The second reason that underlies back pain in pregnancy is the impact of hormonal changes that occur at this time. The pregnancy hormone relaxin makes your ligaments more elastic, allowing the pelvic bones that form the birth canal to accommodate the baby's head during delivery. Unfortunately, because hormones are carried all round the body in the bloodstream, other ligaments also become looser and you are more at risk of general joint strains, as well as strain to the joints in the spine. (For more information on back pain and pregnancy, see *If You're Pregnant*, see page 130.)

A "RELAXIN" EFFECT
One of the pregnancy hormones, relaxin, which loosens your ligaments, is a key contributor to back pain in pregnancy.

Your Back at Work

Many activities pose a risk to your back, including some sports and occasional leisure pursuits, but because your work is part of your daily routine, a "back unfriendly" occupation poses a high risk of long-term problems unless you take special precautions. Luckily, as you'll find out here, there's plenty you can do to avoid problems.

Is my job a back risk? Almost any job could pose a risk to your back if you don't take proper measures to minimize potential sources of trouble. Most people would recognize that heavy manual work could lead to back injuries (for advice, see *Lifting Safely*, page 153), but some jobs that many people consider totally safe, can actually lead to back trouble. Let's look at the reasons why certain jobs present a risk to back health.

Desk work Any job that involves sitting down for hours at a time, particularly if the position is unvarying, is likely to lead to pressure on the disks between the vertebrae. In a sitting position the action of the iliopsoas muscle (page 19) exerts a continuous pressure on the vertebrae in your lower back. The increased pressure in a sitting position raises the risk of the disk moving out of place or losing the soft, cushiony material inside (page 16). It also reduces the space between the vertebrae, leading to an increased likelihood of facet joint problems (page 17). What's more, if your sitting posture isn't good, there's also a risk that the damage will be long term.

How to reduce your risk:
- Take frequent breaks to walk and stretch.
- Adjust your sitting posture (page 156).
- Check that your chair and desk are at a suitable height and that your chair back is angled correctly (page 156).

Driving jobs Any job that involves long periods behind the wheel involves a risk to back health. Some of these are the same as for any other sedentary work, principally disk compression. Perhaps surprisingly, the backs of those who drive cars are more at risk than those who drive trucks, buses, and other large vehicles for a living. This is because the angled position that many car drivers adopt involves a greater strain on the back than the more upright posture of a truck driver. When you are tilted back, too much of the driver's weight is placed on the lower back. In an upright position much of your weight is supported by your thighs. Unfortunately, the constant vibration of driving has a damaging effect on the spine in all types of vehicle.

It's also worth mentioning the risk of whiplash injuries. These most commonly occur as a result of motor vehicle accidents in which there is an impact either from the front or behind. Whiplash injuries (see also *Accidents and Injuries*, page 29) can cause back, neck, and shoulder pain that may persist for several months. What's more, the kinds of impact that cause whiplash may occasionally cause more serious spinal damage.

How to reduce your risk:

- Whether a driver or a passenger, always have a headrest in position to prevent the neck from jerking backward in a collision.
- See page 157 for tips on reducing back strain in a car.

Standing jobs A large number of jobs can involve long periods of standing. These include retail work, security, restaurant and bar work, and many others. The back risk in this type of work is that tiredness can lead to poor posture, which in turn can create stresses on your spine and in the surrounding muscles. (For more about the importance of good posture, see *Take the Right Posture*, page 148.)

How to reduce your risk:

- Walk about whenever you can.
- If possible, stand with one foot up on a stool or footrail. It takes a lot of stress off the low back. Alternate the foot you rest periodically.
- Do stretching exercises every hour or so.
- Lie down, if practical, during longer breaks.

Jobs that involve lifting, carrying, and repeated movements We're talking here not just about work that means carrying heavy loads, but jobs that involve repeatedly carrying lighter loads (for example, waiting tables) or lifting and twisting (supermarket checkout work, for instance, or nursing and house-cleaning).

Day after day, week after week, you can perform the same movement without a problem, then one day you feel your back "go." This is because regular strain on the back along with poor posture can damage the disks over time, so that, eventually, even a minor stress can cause a disk to rupture or prolapse. Other possible problems related

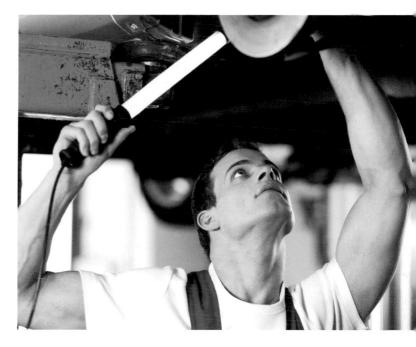

to regular stress include inflammation of the facet joints and over-stretching of the supporting ligaments—both of which can weaken the whole structure, and allow the vertebrae to be nudged out of alignment.

IT'S A STRAIN
Jobs that involve moving your arms over your head, especially when under strain, can easily lead to back trouble.

How to reduce your risk:

- Avoid lifting and twisting at the same time. Always lift a load straight in front of you.
- Rest frequently if carrying out a task that involves repeating the same movement for an extended period of time.
- Always follow the lifting and carrying advice on page 153 even for light loads.

Types of Back Pain

For most people, understanding how and why their backs hurt is a key part of finding a solution that works for them. On the following pages you will learn how certain stimuli are registered and felt as pain—something you need to know as you and your doctor discuss possible treatments.

The pathways of pain When we feel pain, the brain is interpreting a signal from elsewhere in the body that has been transmitted through peripheral nerves and the spinal cord from an area of the body that has been damaged. It is important to realize that pain does not always indicate new damage, but may be a response to a problem that occurred some time ago. It may also occur without obvious physical cause, and may reflect anxiety or fear.

The "messengers" that carry pain signals are chemicals called neurotransmitters that are produced in nerve fiber cells. Neurotransmitters pass the message from cell to cell to the brain, which "translates" the signal so that we feel pain.

The Gate The "Gate Theory of Pain" is one way many scientists explain the transmission of pain signals. It's a key concept in pain management

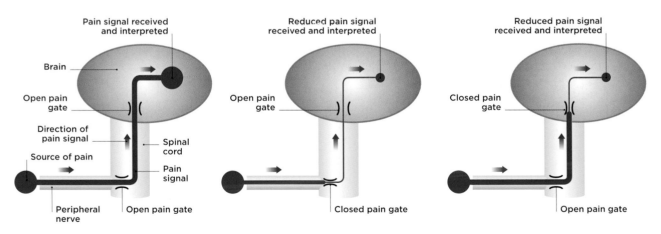

NO PAIN RELIEF
Following an injury or other painful stimulus, the pain signal travels along a peripheral nerve and is transmitted via the spinal cord to the brain where it is interpreted as pain.

PAIN RELIEF AT THE SPINAL CORD
Additional nerve stimulation, such as massage or TENS, may block the pain gate at the spinal cord, reducing the intensity of pain signals reaching the brain.

PAIN RELIEF IN THE BRAIN
Chemicals in the brain—endorphins—released in response to fear or other stimuli can close the pain gate in the brain. Some painkilling drugs also work in this way.

Fiber Facts ▸▸

There are two types of nerve fiber involved in the transmission of pain: A-fibers and C-fibers.

A-fibers are covered with a sheath of fatty material called myelin that enables nerve impulses to travel through them exceptionally rapidly. These are the fibers that transmit signals arising from pressure or injury such as a cut, burn, or torn muscle. They prompt sharp, intense pain.

C-fibers do not have a myelin sheath. They carry slower signals that warn of disease or damage within the body and produce sensations of aching or soreness.

Most back pain is conveyed along C-fibers and can be interrupted by stimulation of the nearby A-fibers—by rubbing, for example—which produces at least temporary pain relief.

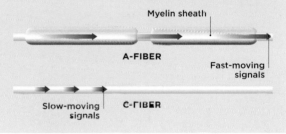

because by understanding how pain is transmitted, you can learn how to interrupt its signals and so relieve it.

Here's the way scientists think it works (see also the diagrams, left): Nerve signals from the pain site pass through a number of junctions or "gates" on their way to the brain. The first of these is where the peripheral nerves join the spinal cord. If too many signals try to get through the gate, priority is given to the signals that travel along what doctors call "A-fibers" (see above). A-fibers are like the "emergency vehicles only" lane on a freeway or highway—and nobody gets in their way. Once the A-fiber signals have gotten through, however, everyday pain signals that travel along "C-fibers"—like the regular lanes most of us travel on highways—are allowed to go through that gate.

Gates further along the pain transmission path to and through the brain work on a different principle: they can be closed by the action of brain chemicals called endorphins. Endorphins, which can block pain, are released in response to fear, physical activity, relaxation, and sleep. Many painkilling medications work by mimicking their actions in the brain. (See also *Drug Treatment*, page 204.)

Acute or chronic? Doctors usually divide back pain into two broad categories—acute and chronic.

Back pain that comes on suddenly is termed "acute." Acute pain can vary widely—from a dull ache to severe pain that prevents movement. This type of pain usually gets better within about six weeks. It's typically caused by strain or injury arising from a specific event, such as lifting an unusually heavy weight. But acute pain can also occur as a consequence of the sudden worsening of a long-term (chronic) problem.

Chronic back pain is persistent and long-term—usually lasting longer than six weeks. The pain may be present all the time, but often consists of recurrent periods of mild, moderate, or severe pain. Chronic pain can arise from a wide variety of conditions that cause back problems, including various forms of arthritis, postural or occupational problems, spinal curvatures, and muscle imbalances.

Whether a pain is acute or chronic can affect the urgency of the action you need to take. (For more information on seeking help, see *How Do I Know What's Wrong?*, page 38.)

Is It All in Your Head? ▸▸

Many people believe that unless there is a verifiable physical cause for pain, it can be dismissed as imaginary. But modern pain specialists recognize that our mental state can have a profound effect on how we experience pain. And since all pain is interpreted in the brain, pain arising from psychological causes is no less real or less painful than discomfort from a physical injury.

In practice, most pain has both a physical and a psychological aspect. One person's minor twinge arising from a back strain is another person's excruciating agony—necessitating a different treatment for each.

What's more, an initial examination that doesn't reveal an immediate physical cause for back pain doesn't mean that there isn't a physical problem. It may be that further diagnostic tests and examinations are needed to discover the source of the trouble.

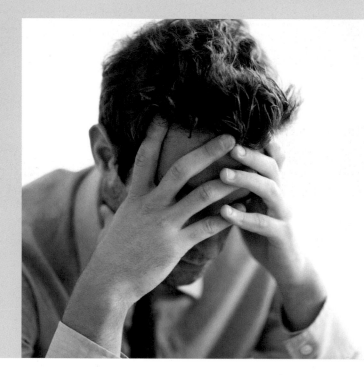

Where's the problem? Since nerves that serve all areas of the body originate in the spinal cord, damage or disease in the spine can contribute to your pain by compressing or inflaming a peripheral nerve as it joins the spinal cord, or the root of a nerve as it emerges from the spinal cord and makes its way between the vertebrae to the part of your body that it serves.

Either way, a damaged or diseased spine can cause symptoms that the brain interprets as coming from an area served by that nerve. An injury to one of the cervical (neck) vertebrae, for example, can cause pain that appears to come from the arm. Or compression of the lumbar (lower back) vertebrae can cause shooting pains down the back of a leg (sciatica). But referred pain, as this is called, can also cause pain that comes from elsewhere in the body, to be "felt" in the brain as coming from the back.

SOURCES OF REFERRED PAIN
Some common causes of referred pain in the back are listed in the table below.

Back Pain That's Not in the Back ▸▸

Disorder	Type of back pain
Heart attack or angina	May be felt as pain in the back, as well as the chest and/or arm
Gall bladder problems	May be felt as pain just below the shoulder blade
Lung infection	May be felt as mid-back pain
Stomach ulcer or cancer	May be felt as pain between the shoulder blades
Inflammation of the pancreas	May be felt as intermittent mid-back pain
Menstrual cramps or inflammation of the uterus	May be felt as low-back pain

The Language of Pain ▸▸

Here are some simple explanations of the terms you may hear doctors use in relation to pain:

- **Analgesia** The relief of pain. Painkilling medications are often called analgesics.

- **Central pain** Pain that originates from a problem in the central nervous system (brain and spinal cord).

- **Neuritis** Inflammation of a nerve.

- **Neurogenic pain** Pain that originates in any part of the nervous system.

- **Neuropathy** Disease or disturbance in the functioning of a nerve.

- **Pain threshold** The degree of pain that causes it to be noticed by the affected person.

- **Radiculopathy** Pinched nerve at the spinal column—for example, brachialgia and sciatica.

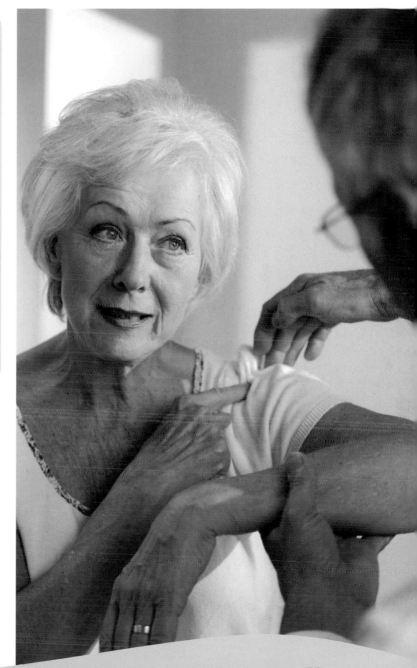

PAIN IN THE ARM
Examination by a doctor will reveal whether the pain you feel in your arm has its origins in your back or elsewhere.

Measuring pain

Pain is not always easy to measure or evaluate. But researchers at the University of Aberdeen, Scotland, devised a simple questionnaire to help those with low-back pain assess the severity of their pain. By filling out the questionnaire at the start of treatment, and periodically during your treatment program, you can actually see for yourself how your symptoms are improving day by day. You can download the questionnaire from the Centre for Evidence Based on Physiotherapy (www.cebp.nl).

How Do I Know What's Wrong?

Pain is generally either acute (sudden, often severe) or chronic (recurrent or long-term). Either type can need expert care and occasionally it is vital to seek emergency help. Use the information here to help you understand what might be wrong, but do not delay in consulting your doctor. Only a physician can distinguish between a minor, passing issue and something more serious.

Get Help ▸▸

Following an injury, if pain is severe or you have numbness, tingling, or weakness in your arms or legs or if you lose control of bowel or bladder (or are unable to pass urine or move your bowels), have someone call 911 or your local emergency services, or call them yourself. Otherwise, do not move your back or neck (or allow anyone who is not a paramedic to move you). Keep still and ask others to keep you warm until help arrives.

Look for the description on these pages that most closely fits your case to get an insight into the possible cause of your trouble. Remember, you should always seek medical help if you are in any doubt about the cause of your symptoms, especially if chronic pain starts to become worse. Whatever the suspected reason for your problem, if pain is significant, unusual, or continues to worsen, don't hesitate to see your physician.

SUDDEN-ONSET BACK PAIN

This is sudden, often severe pain that comes on following an accident or other event that put your back under unusual strain. It may also occur for no apparent reason.

After a fall or other injury In all but the most minor bumps and knocks, treat any injury to the back as potentially serious. There is a possibility of damage that could cause permanent disability if not treated by a doctor. Even apparently minor injuries can cause serious conditions and require immediate medical assessment.

■ **Action advice** In all cases call your family physician without delay. Check the symptoms described under *Get Help* (left) and take appropriate action.

After lifting and/or twisting A sudden twist, especially under strain, can cause the facet joints (page 16) to be pushed out of alignment so that the joint becomes swollen and inflamed and the surrounding muscles go into spasm. Such movements can also cause a disk between the spine's vertebrae to protrude from the joint space, putting pressure on the spinal cord (see page 116).

■ **Action advice** If you have back pain with impaired sensation or movement of the arms or legs, call your physician at once. Subject to the go-ahead from your physician, try the self-help advice on page 214. The sciatica relief position and the McKenzie exercise (page 138) may also give relief.

If you also have pain in the arms or shoulders, this may be brachialgia (page 82).

- **Action advice** Call your physician. Subject to your physician's advice, follow the self-help tips on page 214. Wear a soft collar to support the neck and relax the neck muscles for the first few days.

If you also have pain down the back of the legs, this is likely to be sciatica (page 118).

- **Action advice** After checking with your physician, lie on your back with a pillow under your knees for 24 hours if pain is extreme, but try to get up and move around as soon as possible. You may find the tips on page 214 help to relieve symptoms. Consult your physician again if pain persists or becomes worse.

GRADUAL ONSET SEVERE BACK PAIN

This advice applies to pain that has come on gradually over the past few days and is now severe. If you are also experiencing additional symptoms such as tiredness, weight loss, a fever, and pain

Nerve Pain ▸▸

Nerves can be pinched or damaged either within the spinal column or as they exit through the vertebral openings. In the cervical vertebrae in the neck, such damage can cause headaches and pain, pins and needles, and numbness in the shoulder and down the arm; in the thoracic vertebrae it can cause pain around the rib cage and on deep breathing, sneezing, or laughing; and in the lumbar and sacral vertebrae it can cause pain, pins and needles, and numbness in the buttocks and down the legs. (See also *Where's the problem*, page 36.)

Meningitis Alert ▸▸

One of the common symptoms of meningitis, a potentially fatal and fast-moving condition, is a stiff neck. It is vital that you rule out meningitis if you have one, so check for other common symptoms that may have developed over the last few hours or days, such as a headache, fever, nausea and vomiting, and an aversion to bright lights. A rash that does not fade when pressed with a glass can also be a symptom of meningitis but is not always present.

If you are in any doubt whatsoever about your condition, call your family physician or local emergency services immediately.

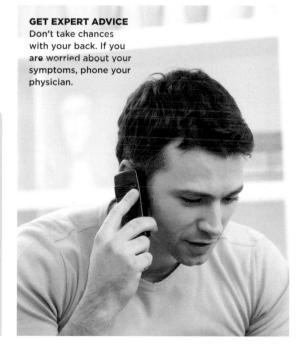

GET EXPERT ADVICE Don't take chances with your back. If you are worried about your symptoms, phone your physician.

at rest, you may have an infection or a non-spinal cause for your symptoms. You should see your family physician without delay.

If you are also unable to control your bladder or bowels (including inability to pass urine or move your bowels) or have numbness around your buttocks, the chance of a serious condition of the spinal cord (see page 50) needs to be ruled out.

- **Action advice** Get emergency help (or go to the emergency room) as soon as possible.

If you also have pain in the legs, your back pain may be the result of sciatica (page 118) or a reduction in the blood supply to the legs.

- **Action advice** See your family physician for expert diagnosis.

Gradual onset pain between the lower back and the top of buttocks, may be the result of sacroiliac joint inflammation (page 124) or ankylosing spondylitis (page 66), or in some cases, having legs of unequal length. This type of back pain is also common among pregnant women (see page 130).

- **Action advice** Be sure to see your family physician for a firm diagnosis and appropriate treatment recommendations.

CHRONIC BACK PAIN

If you experience recurrent or long-term back pain that is not so severe as to be incapacitating, but nonetheless restricts normal activities, you can be said to suffer from chronic back pain. The most common cause is poor posture, but bad lifting techniques, sudden strains, and the general wear

WORSE AFTER SITTING
Pain and stiffness that comes on after long periods of sitting, is often the result of poor posture.

and tear of aging can also be a factor. You should consult your doctor if you have any persistent back pain that does not resolve itself, particularly if it is worsening. Common causes of chronic back pain are discussed below.

Be sure to see your doctor if you have any general symptoms, such as fever, chills, unusual weight loss, or night sweats; if you have numbness or weakness in an arm or leg; if you have had any tumors in the past; if your pain is not relieved by lying down; or if you also have pain in an arm or leg.

If your pain comes and goes frequently, but for no apparent reason, the likely causes are stress (page 162), poor posture (page 148), or strain from carrying heavy loads (page 152).

- **Action advice** Consult your family physician for a firm diagnosis. There is additional advice on relaxation, posture, and avoidance of strain on pages 162, 148, and 152 respectively.

If your pain is persistent and becoming worse, and you are an older person, a likely cause is inflammation (page 30). But there is a chance that you have a tumor (page 50) or other condition such as osteoarthritis (page 58) or cervical spondylosis (page 92). If you are a younger person and your pain improves after exercise, ankylosing spondylitis (page 66) could be the cause.

- **Action advice** In all cases of this type of pain, consult your family physician.

If your pain occurs after carrying heavy loads or after unusual activity, muscle spasm, muscle strain, and ligament sprain (page 29) are likely causes.

- **Action advice** Consult your family physician for an expert diagnosis.

If your pain is between the shoulder blades, you may have a muscular imbalance (page 27).

- **Action advice** Consult your family physician, who may refer you to a physical therapist (page 178).

Women and Back Pain ▶▶

Chronic back pain in older women can be caused by osteoporosis (page 68); the condition is much less common in men and younger women. But a variety of gynecological problems, such as endometriosis and fibroids, can also cause chronic pain in the lower back. So any woman who experiences long-term, persistent or recurrent back pain should consult her family physician.

If pain in the middle back persists for long periods and not just after activity, you could have stomach or gall bladder problems.

- **Action advice** See your family physician.

If your pain becomes worse after activity and/ or exposure to cold, osteoarthritis (page 58) or cervical spondylosis (page 92) are possibilities.

- **Action advice** See your family physician.

If your pain becomes worse after sitting or standing for long periods, possible explanations include poor posture (page 148) or muscle problems (page 27).

- **Action advice** Follow the advice given on the specified pages later in the book, but consult your family physician for a firm diagnosis first.

An Expert Assessment

If you decide that it's time to seek professional help, you'll want to know what to expect. Here are some of the basic examinations and tests your doctor may use to make a diagnosis.

Listening The first thing most doctors will do is listen to an account of your symptoms. This may sound obvious, but there will be lots of clues that can be gleaned from detailed information such as exactly what the pain feels like, when it occurs, what makes it worse, and what provides relief.

Looking For many types of back problem, observing your posture and the way you move can provide valuable information to a doctor trying to make a diagnosis. This is likely to be followed up by a closer examination of your back. More specifically, your doctor may do the following (see right):

CHECKING HOW FAR YOU CAN MOVE
Your doctor is likely to ask to observe your range of movement bending forward, twisting, and leaning to each side. How far you can move in each direction can give an indication of the area affected and the severity of the problem.

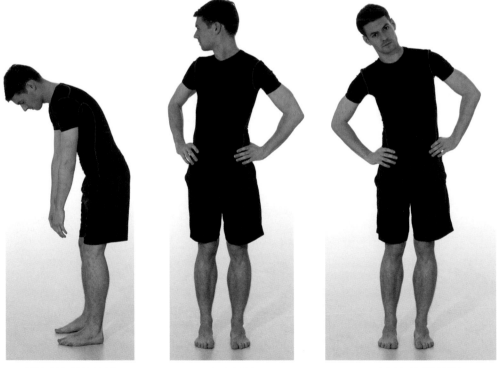

BENDING FORWARD   **TWISTING**   **LEANING TO THE SIDE**

- Examine your spine for any tenderness.
- Assess the range of movement of your spine by asking you to perform certain movements while you are standing and lying down.
- Check your back for any unusual lumps or bumps.
- Check your knee and ankle reflexes, and perform other physical tests for nerve function.

- Examine the range of motion of the hips or shoulders (depending on the region of the back that is affected).

Testing In most cases, the examinations outlined above will be all that's needed to make a preliminary diagnosis. But in many cases, further

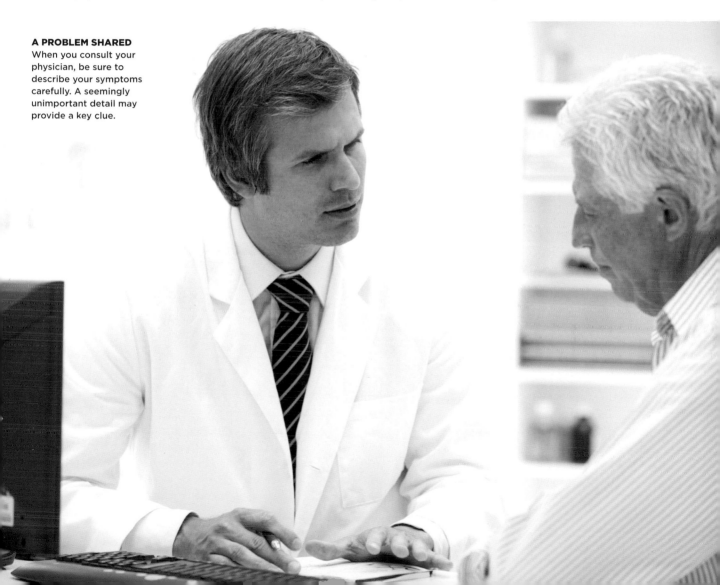

A PROBLEM SHARED
When you consult your physician, be sure to describe your symptoms carefully. A seemingly unimportant detail may provide a key clue.

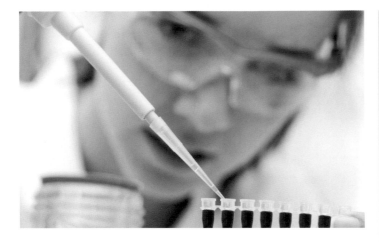

investigations will be needed to confirm this—and these are usually hospital procedures. Depending on your symptoms, one or more of the following tests may be recommended:

IT'S IN THE BLOOD
Analysis of a blood sample can give useful information about your general health as well as that of your back.

- **Blood test** Blood samples may be taken to check for inflammation, infection, or other generalized conditions that may be contributing to your symptoms.
- **Bone density scan** More accurately known as a DXA (dual-energy X-ray absorptiometry) scan, this test tells the doctor if you have or are at risk of bone thinning and therefore fractures (see *Osteoporosis*, page 68).
- **X-ray** A spinal X-ray can reveal a variety of abnormalities in the vertebrae, from fractures to misalignment or joint damage (see *Osteoarthritis*, page 58), but not soft-tissue injuries.
- **Myelography** In this type of imaging, a substance that is opaque on X-ray is injected (under local anesthetic) into the spinal column. A subsequent X-ray reveals the presence of any narrowing of the spinal column (see *Spinal stenosis*, page 116).
- **Diskography** An opaque substance is injected into an intervertebral disk under local anesthetic. The area then shows up on X-ray to reveal disk prolapse or shrinkage.

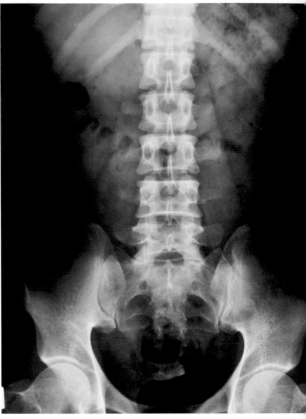

X-RAY VISION
A conventional X-ray image of the spine reveals the condition of the bones. Here we see a normal lumbar spine, sacrum, and pelvis.

- **CT scan** Computerized axial tomography is a type of body scan that integrates numerous X-ray images to provide cross-sectional views of the body. This type of imaging provides detailed information about the bones, which

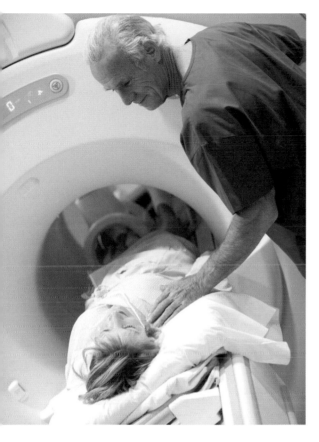

CT SCANNER
Images produced by this system are a useful diagnostic aid for bone-related problems. CT scans can also reveal some soft-tissue abnormalities.

a cylindrical chamber. If this is likely to make you anxious, you may be offered sedative medication to calm your nerves. Since this type of scan can cause any metal inside you to shift, make sure you tell your doctor about any past surgery or metal implants you may have had.

Taking it further Once your doctor has the results of any tests to add to an assessment of your symptoms, a firm diagnosis is likely to be possible and the two of you will decide on the next step.

If no serious underlying cause is found, depending on your condition, your doctor may prescribe medication, advise lifestyle changes, and/or refer you to a physical therapist for appropriate treatment and advice (see page 178). For some conditions, your doctor may even recommend alternative therapies such as massage (see the information on treatment options in Chapter 6).

If your back trouble has been found to be the result of an underlying condition, you may be referred for further medical treatment to an appropriate specialist.

Referral to a back clinic for pain relief injections may also be an option when other measures have failed to alleviate your symptoms.

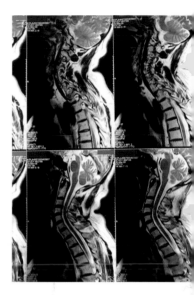

AS SEEN ON MRI
MRI technology produces scans that provide an amazing degree of detail. The vertebrae and spinal cord are clearly visible in this MRI of the neck.

can help in the diagnosis of fractures, disk damage, narrowing of the spinal canal (see *Spinal stenosis*, page 116), osteophyte formation (see *Osteoarthritis*, page 58), and bone damage from tumors (see *Serious But Rare*, page 50).

- **MRI** Magnetic resonance imaging is a type of scanning technology that uses radio waves to provide a detailed picture of the spine, including bones and soft tissues. It can reveal a variety of conditions from disk problems to tumors. While undergoing this type of scan you are enclosed in

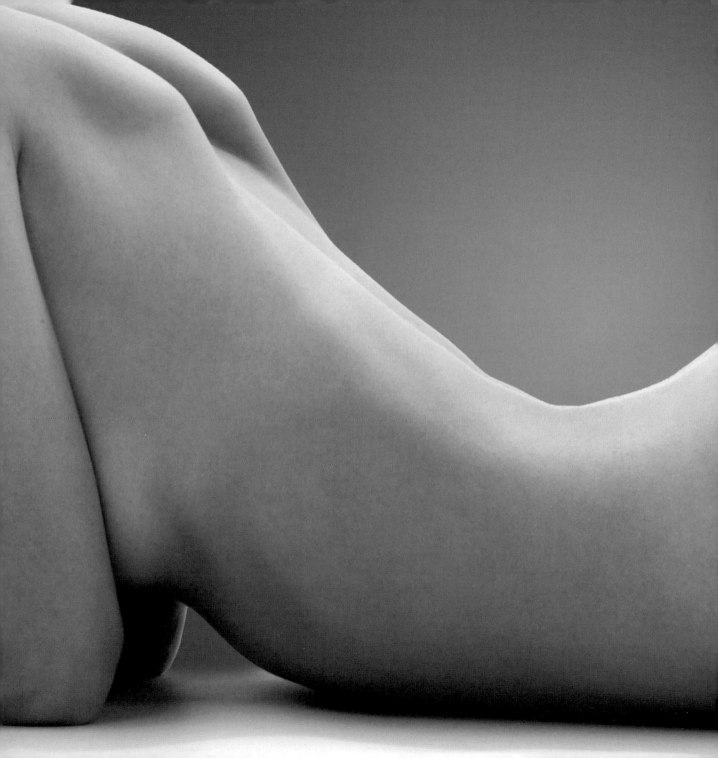

Chapter 2

Conditions Affecting the Whole Back

In this chapter you'll find an overview of the range of back problems that can strike any part of the back or affect the whole spine. These include conditions that can involve many other parts of the body, such as osteoporosis or rheumatoid arthritis, as well as problems specific to the back such as curvatures of the spine.

Challenges to the Whole Back

Your back is a complex structure of interlinked elements. That gives it flexibility and strength. But its complexity also means that a malfunction in one area can have repercussions in another. So sometimes a back problem will affect only one part of the back, and sometimes it will affect the whole thing.

Many back disorders can be the result of problems affecting the spine, or may be caused by more generalized disease. So when you consult your physician about any type of back pain, he or she will consider the possibility that the problem may not be specific to your spine (see also *An Expert Assessment*, page 42).

Misalignment and degeneration Among the conditions that can affect any part of the back are those in which the normal curves of the spine are distorted. Such conditions include abnormal spinal curvatures that can be either congenital or may develop later in life (page 52).

The individual bones of the spine can also be damaged by the degenerative effects of wear and tear on the joints. This is known as osteoarthritis (page 58) and can affect almost any of the hardworking joints in the body over time. Some degree of osteoarthritis is almost universal in older people, although this may be symptomless.

Another category of whole-back disorders includes those in which the bones of the spine—along with other bones in the body—become less dense and therefore more prone to crumbling and fracture. Osteoporosis, the best known of these (page 68), is a major cause of back pain among older people.

Inflammation and infection Some whole-back disorders are part of a generalized inflammatory condition affecting several other body systems. This group of conditions includes the autoimmune diseases—conditions in which the body's natural defense mechanism turns on its own tissues, as in rheumatoid arthritis (page 62) and ankylosing spondylitis (page 66)—and causes widespread inflammation and often disabling pain. Multiple sclerosis (page 51) is another autoimmune disorder—one that affects nerve transmission throughout the body and which can affect the back.

In rare cases the space between the vertebrae in any part of the back may be subject to infection by bacteria. Such infections are termed "discitis." In this condition the germs are usually transmitted to the back from another part of the body via the bloodstream. Occasionally bacteria may be introduced into the spinal area as a result of a surgical procedure.

Pressure on the spinal cord A number of conditions can create pressure on the spinal cord or impinge upon it in other ways, which causes persistent pain and often affects the functioning of this main nerve pathway of the body. Spinal stroke and benign and malignant tumors (see page 50) are among the main causes of spinal cord problems.

BACK TO HEALTH
Some back problems
are the result of a more
generalized disorder for
which treatment by a team
of health professionals may
be required.

SERIOUS BUT RARE

A group of disorders that can affect any part of the spine—and sometimes other parts of the body—include some potentially serious problems, but which are also thankfully rare. Within this category the principal conditions are spinal stroke, spinal tumors, and multiple sclerosis.

Spinal stroke Most people associate a stroke with a problem that affects the brain, but stroke can affect your spinal cord, too. Fortunately, spinal stroke is rare, affecting some 12 in every 100,000 people in America each year at an average age of 52. A "stroke," also called a "spinal cord infarction" when your spinal cord is involved, is an incident in which a blood vessel and its surrounding tissues are damaged either by a lack of oxygen-carrying blood, as a result of a blood clot (ischemic stroke) or, less commonly, by a bleed (hemorrhagic stroke) that causes swelling.

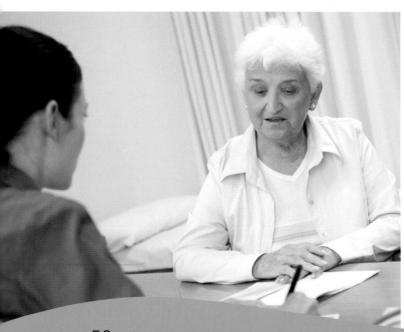

A spinal stroke happens suddenly, and can cause a range of symptoms, depending on which part of the spine is affected. Often there is a sudden paralysis that can progress to cause incontinence, or, if the stroke has occurred in the upper back, breathing may be affected. If you suffer any sudden paralysis or loss of bladder or bowel control, call 911 or your local emergency services without delay.

The most important diagnostic tool in such cases is a magnetic resonance imaging (MRI) scan, allied to a physical examination, blood tests and consideration of your medical history. (For more information on diagnostic tests, see *An Expert Assessment*, page 42.)

Spinal tumors A tumor is an abnormal growth of cells that can be either malignant, in which case it has the capacity to spread to other parts of the body, or benign. Benign tumors do not spread to tissues elsewhere in the body, but they can, depending on their site, cause serious problems, including paralysis. Tumors can start in the spine, in which case they are said to be "primary," but more often they spread to the spine (metastasize) from a tumor elsewhere—"secondary" tumors.

The direct effect of both types of tumor in the back is that the abnormal growth blocks the function of blood vessels, spinal nerves, and spinal bones, depending on its location and nature. As a result, symptoms can vary, but may include a loss of sensation in your arms and legs, back pain that becomes increasingly severe and is not relieved by painkillers, and is unrelieved by lying down. There may also be incontinence or muscle weakness and spasms. If you

THE RIGHT SUPPORT
With any serious condition affecting the back, you'll need to work closely with your physician to get the right treatment.

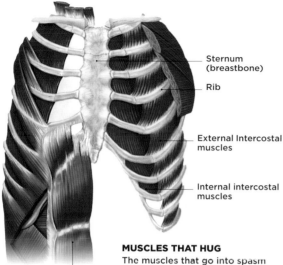

Sternum
(breastbone)

Rib

External Intercostal
muscles

Internal intercostal
muscles

Abdominal
muscles

MUSCLES THAT HUG
The muscles that go into spasm
causing the unpleasant symptom
known as the "MS hug" are the
intercostal muscles.

Barber's Chair Phenomenon ▸▸

Also known as "Lhermitte's sign," this a stabbing sensation, feeling like an electric shock, that runs down your spine from the back of your head when you bend your neck forward—as you would to allow a barber to clip or buzz the hairline on the back of your head. The sensation also affects both arms and legs. Luckily, it normally only lasts for a second or two.

The cause is usually pressure on the spinal cord, which, in turn, may be the result of multiple sclerosis, cervical spondylosis (page 92), a prolapsed disk (page 116), a tumor, or even a deficiency of vitamin B12.

Consult your family physician immediately if you experience a pain such as this.

experience any such symptoms, consult your family physician immediately, because any damage caused can become permanent if you delay. The onset of persistent back pain in anyone who has had cancer in the past should also be brought to a physician's attention promptly.

Diagnosis is by means of a physical examination, followed by X-rays, MRI scans, blood tests, and an examination of cerebrospinal fluid (CSF).

Multiple sclerosis This condition, commonly referred to as MS, affects some 300,000 people in America, and around twice as many women as men. It is an autoimmune disorder, normally striking between the ages of 20 and 40, in which the myelin sheath that surrounds nerves becomes damaged, affecting the transmission of electrical nerve signals. Unfortunately, the condition becomes progressively

worse, although this can happen very gradually and there are often periods of remission, when symptoms do not increase in severity.

MS can affect many different areas of the body, but one of them is the spinal cord, and pain in the lower back is a common symptom. You may also experience the Barber's Chair phenomenon (see above). A specific symptom is the "MS hug," or "MS girdle," in which those affected feel a burning, crushing pain around their whole upper torso. This is because the intercostal muscles (the muscles between each rib) have gone into spasm. Contact your doctor promptly if you experience such a problem. The MS hug can be relieved by muscle relaxants and painkillers (page 204).

Spinal Curvatures

There are three types of spinal curvature: kyphosis, in which the spine of the upper back tilts forward; scoliosis, in which the spine curves either to the right or the left; and lordosis, when the lower back arches outward. Such problems can either be present at birth or develop later.

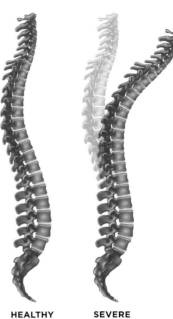

KYPHOSIS

Many people have a small amount of forward rounding of their upper back, but doctors don't usually consider the problem to be kyphosis unless the degree of rounding is greater than 40 degrees. If the cause of kyphosis is long-standing poor posture or an underlying disease process, the degree of rounding is likely to increase and may cause painful symptoms.

KYPHOTIC SPINE
The upper part of a spine affected by kyphosis bends forward, while the natural curve of the lower back is flattened.

HEALTHY SPINE

SEVERE KYPHOSIS

The Hump ▸▸

Dowager's hump is a type of kyphosis often caused by osteoporosis (page 68). It can occur in both sexes, but is more common in elderly women—hence the name.

As the vertebrae are weakened by a reduction in bone density, they become susceptible to compression fractures (see *Osteoporosis*, page 68). Typically the front of the affected vertebrae collapse into a wedge shape and tip forward. This creates a forward-stooping posture and a hunched back. When advanced, the stooping posture may cause tiredness and may inhibit breathing. The exercises opposite help to minimize problems in many cases.

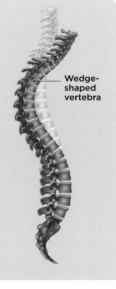

Wedge-shaped vertebra

Symptoms When kyphosis is severe, symptoms may include not just a rounded back but also backache and some breathing difficulties. This last symptom is because the forward tilt of the spine pushes the ribs in toward the lungs and constricts their ability to expand.

What causes kyphosis? When a curvature is present at birth, it's likely that it's been caused by a rare developmental problem that fused or distorted the baby's vertebrae. Kyphosis may also develop during adolescence, especially in girls, when slouching posture stretches the ligaments that support the spine (page 16). Scheuermann's disease, a condition of unknown cause that runs in families and affects more boys than girls, may have the same effect. When kyphosis develops in adulthood, it is usually due to another condition, though poor posture also plays a part. The culprits may be osteoporosis (page 68), which sometimes leads to a dowager's hump (see opposite); osteoarthritis (page 58); rheumatoid arthritis (page 62); and ankylosing spondylitis (page 66). Occasionally, disorders that affect muscles and connective tissue (page 18) or tumors (page 50) may also be responsible.

Prevention Good posture is vitally important, especially during late childhood and adolescence, so encourage your children to adopt a correct posture. For adults, practicing Alexander Technique and Pilates exercises may be useful. If you think you're developing kyphosis, consult your doctor. If there is no underlying cause, the exercises (right) may help. But check with your doctor first.

Figuring out what's wrong Your doctor is likely to ask you to carry out a series of movements while viewing your spine from the side. He or she may ask for an X-ray to check for degenerative changes in your vertebrae and may also conduct tests to check whether kyphosis is affecting your breathing.

Fixing the problem In children and adolescents with Scheuermann's disease a brace is normally fitted. This does not restrict movement as much as you might think. If this doesn't fix the problem, surgery might be necessary to fuse vertebrae (page 210) and reduce the curvature. For other types of kyphosis in young people, an exercise program will be advised. In adults, the underlying cause of kyphosis will be addressed. Physical therapy (page 178), an exercise program, and other therapies such as osteopathy (page 182) may also be recommended (see *What Might Work?*, page 176). Surgery is the last resort.

Exercises for Kyphosis ▸▸

Be sure to check the cautions on page 10 before you try either of these exercises.

Shoulder-blade squeeze
Sit on a stool or low-backed chair that won't restrict your arm movement. Tuck your chin into your chest. While keeping your chest raised, pull your shoulder blades together to bring your elbows back. Hold for five seconds before resting, then repeat 10 times.

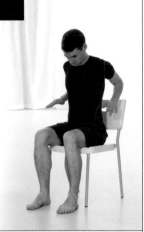

Reverse fly
This exercise calls for some light weights (you can use plastic bottles filled with water) and employs only a small range of motion. Keep your back straight and abs tight throughout.

1 Sit on a chair, grip your weights, and bend over with your head down. Hold the weights next to your ankles with your palms facing inward and keep the head and neck in line with the spine.

2 Raise your arms out to the sides up to shoulder level, squeezing the shoulder blades together as you do. Do not lift your arms any higher than shoulder level. Lower and repeat 10 times.

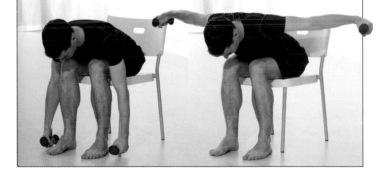

SCOLIOSIS

While kyphosis is an outward and upward curve of the thoracic spine, scoliosis is a spinal curve in a different plane—either to the right or left of a normal spine, as seen from behind. In the classic manifestation of scoliosis, the spine comes to adopt either a C or even an S shape.

Scoliosis affects about twice as many girls as boys, and is most likely to develop any time from early childhood through to adolescence.

Symptoms Other than the curvature of the spine—and sometimes a difference in the apparent height of the shoulders or the hips—there are often no symptoms, though there may be some back pain. In severe cases, the curvature of the spine may affect the movement of the ribs and even the heart, causing shortness of breath and chest pain.

What causes scoliosis? In about 80 percent of cases, the cause of scoliosis is unknown (idiopathic scoliosis), though the condition often runs in families. However, an apparent scoliosis— "apparent" because the spine is, in fact, straight though it appears not to be—can also result from muscular imbalances caused by poor posture, a discrepancy in leg length or overdevelopment of the muscles on one side of the spine, as is seen in some professional tennis players. Another type of scoliosis—generally referred to as functional scoliosis—can develop as a response to a painful stimulus, such as a herniated disk. Or sometimes a severe form of the problem results from a defect in the way that the spinal bones develop in the womb (congenital scoliosis).

Osteoarthritis (page 58) and osteoporosis (page 68) can also cause scoliosis if the damage they cause mostly affects one side of the spine.

Prevention Scoliosis can generally be prevented only when it is caused by muscular imbalances that are created, and then worsened, by poor posture (page 148). In those instances, paying attention to your posture can help stave off the problem. The exercises (opposite) may help in this situation.

Figuring out what's wrong Your physician is likely to ask to observe your naked back as you touch your toes so that he or she can judge whether there is any lack of symmetry. If you are at an age when future growth is possible, the doctor may also take an X-ray of your spine and note your height and weight so that any worsening of the condition can be detected in the future.

Fixing the problem Functional scoliosis is treated by addressing the problem causing the muscular imbalance, often by means of physical therapy (page 178). When scoliosis is idiopathic in a young person, a brace may be fitted to stop the curvature from becoming worse as growth continues. In adults with idiopathic scoliosis a brace has no real benefit. In many cases idiopathic scoliosis corrects

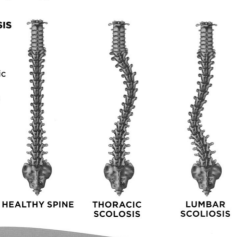

TYPES OF SCOLIOSIS
When the curve is in the upper back's vertebrae, it is described as thoracic scoliosis. When the curve mainly affects the lower back, it is termed lumbar scoliosis.

HEALTHY SPINE

THORACIC SCOLOSIS

LUMBAR SCOLIOSIS

itself over time, especially when its onset was at an early age. Surgery is generally advised for a young person when scoliosis is severe or at any age if there are additional symptoms such as pain, breathing difficulty, or heart problems. Depending on the cause, this may involve the realignment of vertebrae followed by spinal fusion (page 212) to fix them in place, or the removal of osteophytes—bony outgrowths from the vertebrae—formed as a result of osteoarthritis (page 58).

Exercises for Scoliosis Caused by Poor Posture ▸▸

Before doing these exercises, be sure to check with your physician, and read the cautions on page 10.

Diagonal crunch

1 Lie on your back with your knees bent at right angles and place your feet flat on the floor. Place your right hand on the right side of your chest wall and the left hand over your left hip bone.

2 Inhale and then as you exhale tighten your stomach muscles to lift your right side slightly to bring your hands closer together. Repeat five times. Swap hand positions, and lift your left side toward the right five times.

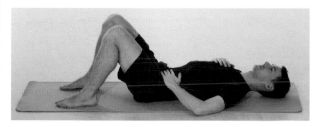

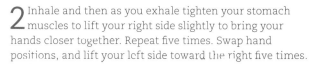

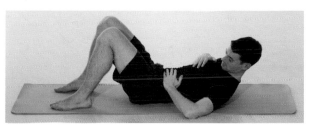

Knee cross-over

Start in the same position as for diagonal crunch (above). Place your hands palm downward at your sides.

1 Cross one leg over the other. Slowly rock your knees as far as possible from side to side, keeping as much of your body in contact with the mat as you can. Try to rock the same amount on each side. Repeat 10 times.

2 Cross the other leg over and repeat the exercise.

HYPERLORDOSIS

As you can see from the diagram of the normal spine on page 14, there is a natural inward curve of the vertebral column in both the neck and lower back. In some people this becomes exaggerated, and in these cases the condition is known as hyperlordosis, also called, in the case of lumbar (lower back) hyperlordosis, "swayback." In the lower back the effect is to push the buttocks upward and outward; in the neck, it makes the head look as if it has been pushed forward.

As well as being ungainly, hyperlordosis can cause pain and limit movement. It also reduces the spine's efficiency as a shock absorber. As a result, even minor injury can cause damage to muscles, ligaments, and vertebrae.

What causes hyperlordosis?

Although hyperlordosis tends to run in families, and in some cases can be present at birth as a result of developmental problems in the womb, most cases are caused by bad posture (page 148). The problem can also arise in later life as a result of a number of other conditions that cause degeneration of the spinal column, such as osteoarthritis (page 58) and osteoporosis (page 68). Injury to the neck or back can also be a contributory factor.

EXAGGERATED CURVES
A spine affected by hyperlordosis typically has a more pronounced curve in the cervical and lumbar regions compared with a healthy spine.

HYPERLORDOSIS

What are the symptoms? Apart from an unnatural and ungainly posture, neither cervical nor lumbar hyperlordosis usually cause any symptoms, other than mild limitation in movement and sometimes mild discomfort. On rare occasions, severe hyperlordosis may cause pressure on nerves as they leave the spinal cord, causing problems at the nerves' roots (page 116).

Prevention The most important preventive measure you can take is to be vigilant about maintaining good posture at all times, and to be ready to make necessary adjustments throughout the day (page 148). Older people also need to take measures to help ward off osteoarthritis (page 58) and osteoporosis (page 68).

Figuring out what's wrong Hyperlordosis is diagnosed by observation and confirmed by X-rays. Your physician will also check on the range of movement of your spine to see if it has become limited in any way.

Fixing the problem Often mild hyperlordosis does not require specific treatment. But if the condition is causing pain, you may be advised to take painkillers—over-the-counter medications such as ibuprofen are often sufficient (see the information on medications starting on page 204).

A physical therapy (page 178) program may be suggested, with the aim of improving your range of movement—examples of some exercises that may be used are given on these pages—and in more severe cases you may also be advised to wear a back brace.

But the emphasis of treatment is on correcting your posture (page 148) and maintaining the improvement by constant vigilance.

Before doing these exercises, be sure to check with your physician and read the cautions on page 10.

Wall sweep

1 Choose a place with a clear area of wall and non-slip floor surface. Stand with your legs shoulder-width apart against a wall, so that your head, upper back, and sacrum are resting against the wall.

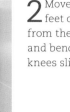

2 Move your feet one foot from the wall and bend your knees slightly.

3 Exhale as you sink down the wall as far as you can—no further than your knees are at right angles—while pressing your lower back into the wall. Hold for a count of 10. Inhale and push yourself up the wall again as you continue to press the small of your back into the wall. Repeat 10 times.

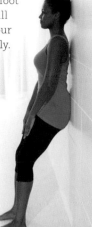

2 Inhale as you lower slowly, pushing the small of your back into the mat throughout. Repeat five times. Repeat the whole exercise raising the other knee and then raise both knees together.

Knee to chest

1 Start by lying on your back with your knees bent at right angles. Support your neck with your hand. Press the small of your back down into the mat. Exhale and raise one knee up toward your chest.

Osteoarthritis

Damage to the joints as a result of aging and overuse is known as osteoarthritis. It is estimated that more than 20 million Americans suffer from osteoarthritis. Many believe that nothing can be done to help restore mobility and relieve pain. But they are wrong. A variety of treatments are available that can, in many cases, improve your quality of life.

The information on these pages focuses on "spinal osteoarthritis," also known as "degenerative arthritis of the spine." Confusingly, doctors may talk of "cervical spondylosis" (page 92) when osteoarthritis affects the vertebrae in the neck region, and "lumbar degenerative disk disease" when the condition affects the lower back.

Symptoms Osteoarthritis usually produces symptoms that develop slowly, often over many years. Pain, as a result of inflammation of the joint lining caused by the rubbing together of bones, is the main symptom. The pain usually becomes worse when stress is placed on the affected joints by activity, and may be made worse by muscle imbalances caused by your body's attempts to protect the joints.

Often osteoarthritis does not produce any symptoms. We know this because most people over 60 can be shown to have osteoarthritic changes on X-rays, but do not report symptoms.

What causes osteoarthritis? There are two main causes: primary and secondary. In the first, which is by far the most common cause, aging is responsible. As you become older, the water content of the cartilage that forms your intervertebral disks diminishes, reducing their size and making them

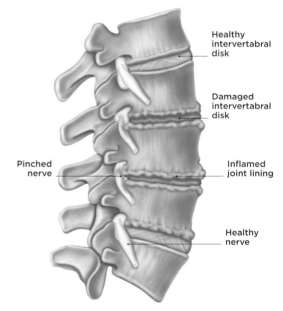

Healthy intervertabral disk

Damaged intervertabral disk

Pinched nerve

Inflamed joint lining

Healthy nerve

OSTEOARTHRITIS IN THE SPINE
Loss of water from the intervertebral disks leads to a reduction in the space between the vertebrae, causing the bones to rub together, causing inflammation and pain.

rough. At the same time, your facet joint capsule (page 16) and the supporting ligaments become thicker and tighter. All of this leads to a narrowing of the space between the vertebrae, with those in the neck and lower back being particularly susceptible. What's more, being overweight adds to the pressure on them. Eventually, bone starts to rub on bone, causing pain, and the intervertebral joints become inflamed. Perhaps in an attempt to protect the joints, bony spurs, called "osteophytes," often form on their margins, though they do not always cause symptoms. These degenerative changes may affect the nerves in the spine.

In secondary osteoarthritis the same process takes place, but the cause can be an injury to a joint, a genetic condition that affects cartilage, diabetes, muscles imbalances in your back or pelvis, or any of a number of other conditions that cause joint inflammation.

Prevention There is a limited amount you can do to prevent osteoarthritis which is caused by years of joint use. And weight-bearing exercise, which makes the condition more likely, is what is recommended as protection against another back problem—osteoporosis (page 68). You need to aim to achieve a balance.

Maintaining a healthy weight (see page 158) and maintaining easy joint movement with non–weight-bearing exercise like swimming are both good strategies to keep osteoarthritis at bay.

Figuring out what's wrong Physicians can generally make a diagnosis on the basis of your symptoms, your medical history, and an examination of your joints. Your doctor may also suggest that you have an X-ray to confirm the diagnosis and to assess the degree of the problem.

What Puts You at Risk? ⯈

Some people are lucky enough to survive into a ripe old age without having any problems with osteoarthritis—so even while the risks increase with age, it is not inevitable that you will have problems. Here's what puts you at risk:

- You are a woman: women are three times more likely than men to develop primary osteoarthritis.
- Your family has a history of the condition.
- You are overweight—even, some say, by as little as 10 pounds (4.5 kg).
- You have suffered an injury or were born with a deformity that has placed abnormal stresses on a joint.
- You get little exercise, and so are losing full mobility in your joints.
- You suffer from a condition, such as diabetes or gout, that can cause cartilage degeneration.
- Overuse—possibly caused by a long working life involving lifting.

WEIGHT WATCH
By keeping an eye on the scales and taking prompt steps to deal with those extra pounds, you can reduce your risk of osteoarthritis.

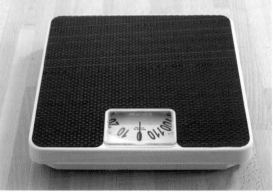

Fixing the problem Over-the-counter painkillers, such as acetaminophen, are often the first line of treatment, while stronger nonsteroidal anti-inflammatory drugs (NSAIDs) may be prescribed if other medications prove ineffective. (For more information on medications, see page 204.) But the main treatments for osteoarthritis are physical therapy (page 178) and lifestyle modification. Physical therapy, using individually tailored programs, has been shown to significantly reduce pain levels and increase mobility. But lifestyle modification, in particular by reducing your weight and increasing your levels of physical activity, can be equally effective. Just be careful not to overdo

Exercise and Osteoarthritis ▸▸

Exercise is one of the mainstays of treatment for osteoarthritis, because it helps maintain joint mobility. But it's important that you do the correct exercises in the correct way—otherwise you risk making your problem worse.

How do you know which exercises will help? If you have neck problems, say, sitting to stabilize your trunk and then looking over each shoulder in turn (page 97) may be in order; if you have low-back arthritis, you may benefit from doing pelvic tilts (page 134). But much depends on which joints are affected and how much. So ask your doctor or physical therapist (page 178) to help you work out an exercise program that is right for you.

Follow the golden rules Your professional advisers will tell you there are two golden rules when it comes to osteoarthritis exercises: start slowly and build up the intensity and frequency of each exercise gradually; second, never try to push through your pain, because doing so can be dangerously counter-productive. Remember, for those with osteoarthritis, "No pain, no gain" is simply not true.

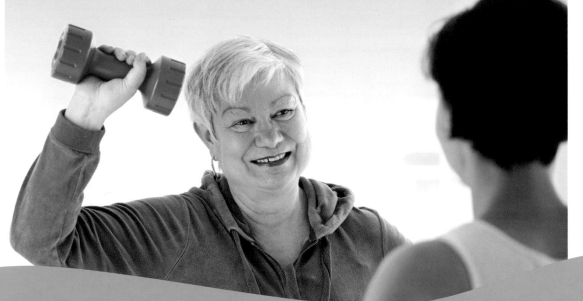

No Excuses! ▸▸

Analysis of the skeletons of mummies found in the tombs of the ancient Egyptian pharaohs has revealed than many of them suffered from debilitating arthritis—even from as early as their mid 40s. This may be because of the close family links between them all and the likely genetic basis of the condition.

One such sufferer was the legendary Ramesses II, known as "the Great," who ruled Egypt for more than 66 years. He probably started to suffer from arthritis in mid-life, but is thought to have been 96 when he died. And it was an eventful life: he led an army of more than 100,000 men to numerous victories; he founded cities, built splendid tombs and monuments; and is thought to have fathered more than 90 children. Obviously, arthritis did not slow him down!

The Claw of the Devil? ▸▸

You might think that a plant variously known as "Devil's claw," the "Grapple plant," and the "Wood spider" should be avoided—but you could be wrong. And not just because the "claws" are just tiny hooks that cover the fruit of this southern African native species.

A number of research studies have shown that taking supplements derived from Devil's claw roots can be as effective as many conventional medications in relieving pain and reducing symptoms in osteoarthritis suffers, including those whose neck or lower back are affected. They also give rise to fewer side effects.

But a word of caution Consult your physician before trying Devil's claw, because it can interact with other medications (blood-thinning agents, in particular) and may be inappropriate if you suffer from some other conditions. Also, no long-term safety information is available. It should not be taken during pregnancy or while you are breastfeeding.

it; gentle swimming and water aerobics are ideal activities. Carefully supervised yoga (page 196) with a trained teacher may also be of benefit. Acupuncture (page 198) has been reported to relieve symptoms for some people.

There is some debate about whether products containing glucosamine and chondroitin, both of which are constituents of cartilage, are effective. Some reports suggest that they may be useful but most doctors will tell you that these supplements produce little benefit.

If all else fails, surgery (page 210) may be considered, depending on the type of joint involved and its condition. But surgery isn't suitable for everyone, and there are significant risks associated with all types of spinal surgery. Be sure to discuss your options carefully with your healthcare team.

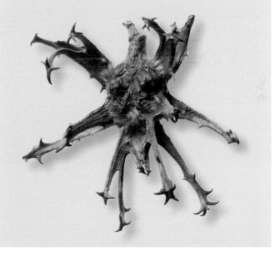

Rheumatoid Arthritis

Rheumatoid arthritis (RA) is a "rheumatic disease," that can affect the organs and systems of the whole body. It is a serious, long-term, and progressive condition, but one in which there are often periods in which the disease does not cause any symptoms. Fortunately, modern treatment can prolong these symptom-free periods and slow the disease progress.

Rheumatoid arthritis is an autoimmune condition, in which the body's defense mechanism attacks its own tissues. It affects about 1.3 million Americans, and three times more women than men have the condition. It can strike at any stage of life, but it usually becomes apparent between ages 40 and 60.

RA is thought to cost the American healthcare system about $39 billion a year. Not surprisingly, research into the condition is a high priority and this work is producing promising results.

Symptoms In RA, joints lubricated by synovial fluid become inflamed—and a large number of the joints in your body, including the facet joints of the vertebrae, are synovial. (See page 16 for more information about the joints of the spine.) This inflammation leads to a reduction in mobility and damage to bones and cartilage. In the spine, the cervical (neck) vertebrae are most commonly affected by this condition.

The symptoms of RA tend to come and go, often being inactive for months or even years. This makes the condition difficult to diagnose early. The hands and wrists are often the first to be affected, leading over time to severe deformities.

The disease often affects the cervical vertebrae, leading to pain at the base of the neck as the

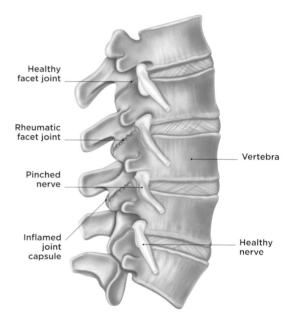

Healthy facet joint

Rheumatic facet joint

Pinched nerve

Inflamed joint capsule

Vertebra

Healthy nerve

JOINT DAMAGE
Rheumatoid arthritis involves pain and swelling of the synovial (fluid-lubricated) joints in the body, including those of the spine.

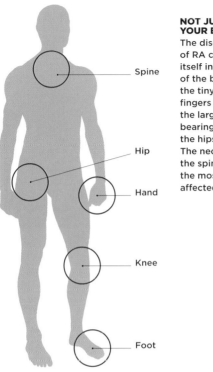

The disease process of RA can manifest itself in many areas of the body, from the tiny joints in the fingers and toes to the large weight-bearing joints of the hips and knees. The neck region of the spine is among the most commonly affected.

Spine

Hip

Hand

Knee

Foot

vertebrae become unable to support the weight of the skull, and so slip a bit, leading to deformities and the serious risk of spinal cord compression at the base of the skull.

Compression in other areas of the spine may first become apparent if your gait starts to change. You may also experience weakness and problems in keeping your balance. When the condition is active, there is muscle and joint stiffness, frequently accompanied by tiredness, a raised temperature, and a loss of appetite.

RA can also affect other organs and systems of the body, such as the lungs, kidneys, heart, liver ("Felty's syndrome"), and the eyes ("Sjögren's syndrome"), which often become dry and inflamed.

The Supplement Debate ▸▸

Many people advocate dietary supplements to combat rheumatoid arthritis, but unfortunately their efficacy has not been proved. Omega-3 fish oil supplements, for example, are often suggested. But though they can be shown to have anti-inflammatory effects in the laboratory there is no proof that they produce the same effects in the body. The same goes for cartilage boosters, such as glucosamine and chondroitin.

Which nutrients are helpful? While supplements may not have been proved to slow the progress of the disease, it is possible that they may reduce symptoms—and some nutrients will also improve your general health. In particular, it may be helpful to increase your intake of foods high in antioxidants—nutrients that counter the action of the inflammatory substances known as free radicals. Foods high in antioxidants include apples, apricots, beans, berries, broccoli, carrots, leeks, onions, and whole grains. It's also a good idea to have plenty of omega-3 rich oily fish, such as salmon, herring, and sardines in your diet, too. And apricots, beets, carrots, paprika, pumpkin, and sweet potato will boost your levels of beta-carotene, an antioxidant that research suggests is reduced in those with RA. Be sure to consult your physician before taking nutritional supplements or making changes to your diet.

GO FISH
Oily fish, such as sardines, are a rich source of omega-3 essential fatty acids, which are thought to counter inflammation.

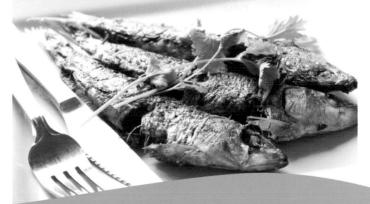

What causes rheumatoid arthritis? Nobody knows for sure. What is clear is that a family history of RA predisposes to it, and there is strong evidence that cigarette smoking, stress, and obesity are all risk factors. There is also some evidence that vitamin D deficiency, low estrogen levels, and low levels of antioxidants may be involved—though the extent of this association has not been proved.

It is thought that, especially when risk factors are present, a viral or bacterial infection may trigger an autoimmune response in which your body's defensive immune system starts to target your body's own tissues.

Prevention The onset of RA can be made less likely, and the severity of its symptoms reduced, if you avoid risk factors. So:

- Stay away from tobacco smoke.
- Make sure you get sufficient levels of vitamin D and antioxidants, either in your diet, as supplements, or by regular exposure to sunlight.

In order to slow the condition's progress, if you have already been diagnosed with RA, and to help stay in remission, do the above—but also:

- Exercise to maintain and improve your mobility.
- Lose weight, if you are overweight or obese, to avoid putting further strain on your joints (see *Lighten Up*, page 158).
- Consider dietary measures (see the panel on supplements on page 63).

Figuring out what's wrong A doctor may first suspect RA after looking at your joints to see whether they are swollen, twisted in any way, or tender; stiffness (characteristically in the morning) and decreasing mobility are also key indicators. The relative numbers of small and large joints affected are an important part of the diagnosis. Blood samples are also taken. In about 80 percent of people who have RA, an antibody—that is, a protein that destroys material identified as foreign—called "rheumatic factor" is found, but some people who have this antibody in their blood do not have RA.

Fixing the problem The earlier a diagnosis is made and treatment can start the better in order to reduce the risk of irreversible joint damage.

The pain of RA can be relieved by medication (page 204), including nonsteroidal anti-inflammatory drugs (NSAIDs) and acetaminophen. Physical therapists (page 178) can provide an individually tailored program to help maintain your joint mobility and improve muscle strength.

Gold-standard Treatment ▸▸

Gold salts—a group of DMARDs—have been used medicinally for more than 200 years, although their use as a treatment for RA fell out of fashion in the 1980s. In 1997 a research project undertaken by the Cochrane Institute found that gold injections can be an effective treatment for RA since they appear to reduce joint inflammation and slow the condition's progress. That is, if patients can withstand the side effects, such as gastrointestinal irritation, and the weekly injections at the start of the treatment program.

Can I go for gold? Unfortunately, much of the gold given is excreted from the body within a short time, the treatment takes three to six months to take effect, and it does not work on everyone. The side effects mean that around 30 percent of patients cannot continue with treatment. One rare side effect of long-term use is that your skin turns bluish. But ask your doctor; gold might work for you.

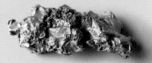

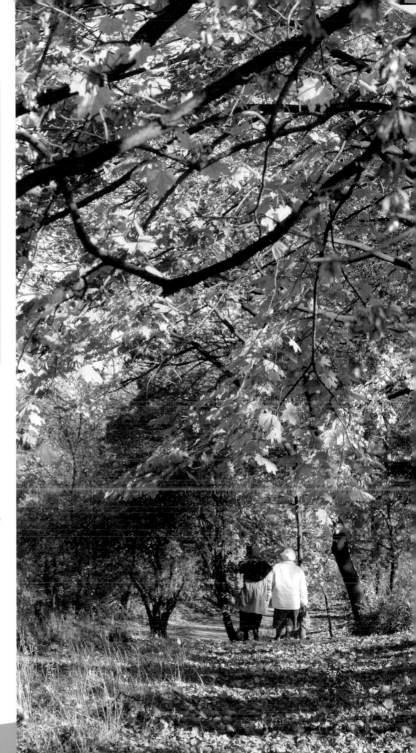

Women at Risk ▸▸

The incidence of RA in both men and women had been declining for more than 40 years until around 1995. But then it started to increase by 2.5 percent a year over the next decade—but only in women. In men, its incidence continued to decrease by 0.5 percent a year.

Why? Nobody knows for sure, but there are some interesting pointers. First, smoking rates have declined less in women than in men—and smoking is a risk factor for RA. Secondly, vitamin D deficiency, also thought to be linked to the condition, is more prevalent in women. Thirdly, and more speculatively, it is thought that the low dosage of estrogen in the modern oral contraceptives has a less protective effect than the older, higher-dosage contraceptive pill.

Massage therapy (page 186), acupuncture (page 198), and TENS (page 202) may provide relief of symptoms. It may also be helpful to consult an occupational therapist for help with coping with household chores and prolonging your working life. Surgery (page 210) to help increase mobility may be considered.

The main treatment of the condition itself consists of "disease-modifying antirheumatic drugs" (DMARDs). These have been proved to increase remission times and delay the progress of RA. Physicians now use them in the early stages of the condition, even though they may cause side effects. Other drugs that may be offered include tumor necrosis factor blockers (page 208).

WALK ON
Treatment for RA designed to maintain mobility can often help keep you active and able to enjoy life to the full.

Ankylosing Spondylitis

Also known as "bamboo spine," ankylosing spondylitis is an autoimmune disorder—a condition in which the body's defenses attack its own tissues. The result is chronic inflammation—mainly in the spine—and the vertebrae gradually fuse. Treatment can usually permit you to live a relatively normal life.

Symptoms The condition normally develops when someone is in their 20s or 30s, though in about 5 percent of cases it develops in childhood. More men are affected than women. It usually affects the low back first. The first signs are back pain and stiffness that is often worse in the morning. The symptoms can spread to the upper buttocks, neck, and the rest of the spine. Often additional symptoms such as general tiredness, night sweats, and swelling in other joints follow. In some cases, inflammation also affects the soles of the feet and the Achilles tendon at the back of the calf. Rarely, the eyes, the skin, the heart, and the kidneys can be affected.

These initial symptoms tend to come and go, in varying degrees of severity. But over the years bouts of disease activity can slowly lead to the vertebrae in the affected areas becoming fused.

If not treated, fusion of the vertebrae can severely restrict mobility and lead to a characteristic stooping posture as the thoracic spine curves forward. This distortion of the spine may affect breathing and may scar the lungs.

The spine also becomes brittle and more likely to fracture, especially in the lower part of the neck—even after a seemingly innocuous fall. Any neck pain or change of head position after such an event should be treated as a medical emergency if you have been diagnosed with this condition.

Healthy spine

DISTORTED SPINE
The chronic inflammation that occurs in ankylosing spondylitis causes the ligaments to become bony, which results in fusion of the vertebrae at the base of the spine and a forward-leaning curvature.

Fused vertebrae

What causes ankylosing spondilitis? This is an inherited condition that affects about one in a hundred people. It's thought that factors other than genes may also contribute, because while 7 percent of the population carry the genes involved, the condition only develops in a small proportion.

Neither the causes nor the process by which the condition develops and causes inflammation and spinal fusion are yet fully understood. Continuing research may provide new insights into the causes and treatment of this condition in the future.

Prevention Unfortunately, there are no preventive measures that can guard against the onset of ankylosing spondylitis. If you know the condition runs in your family, be alert for the symptoms and if you suspect you're affected, get a diagnosis as early as possible to improve your chances of avoiding structural damage to the spine.

Figuring out what's wrong The complex and intermittent pattern of the emergence of symptoms in the early stages of the condition can delay diagnosis. But over time a good physician will recognize the range of symptoms and confirm the diagnosis by means of X-rays, blood tests to identify genetic markers, and possibly magnetic resonance imaging (MRI).

Fixing the problem Medications that affect immune system activity are available, but unfortunately many of them have a risk of serious side effects. Drugs such as aspirin and NSAIDs may be tried for pain reduction and their inflammation-reducing effect, but they are not always effective. If they are not, antirheumatic drugs such as methrotrexate and sulfasalazine may be used, though neither of these reduce inflammation in the spine. A newer group of medicines called tumor necrosis factor blockers (TNFs) are often beneficial. Injections of cortisone, a steroid drug, may also be helpful. (For detailed information about drugs and their possible side effects, see page 204.)

Alongside medication, the mainstay of treatment is physical therapy (page 178). Exercise programs that focus on improving posture and strengthening the back muscles are tailored to an individual's needs, depending on how the condition has progressed. Generally, a program will emphasize exercises to improve breathing and spinal flexibility.

Go for the Gold! ▸▸

Two international sporting superstars can attest to the fact that achieving your personal best in a sport—even with ankylosing spondylitis—is far from being a dream.

Rico Brogna, the Major League Baseball first baseman, was diagnosed with the condition in 1991. Yet in 1999 he hit a career-high 24 home runs for the Philadelphia Phillies. He is now an ambassador for the Spondylitis Association of America.

The golfer Ian Woosnam was diagnosed in 1987. Yet in 1991 he won the Masters Tournament at the Augusta National Golf Club, and in the same year spent 50 weeks as World Golf Number 1. In 2006 he was Captain of the victorious European Ryder Cup team in Ireland. He still plays in the European Seniors Tour, though more than 50 years old.

Whatever program is prescribed, you need to stick to it to reduce spinal distortion and maintain mobility. With such treatment, it is possible to enjoy a wide range of physical activities.

It is also important to modify your lifestyle, both at home and in the workplace. You should ensure that you sleep on a firm, level bed, with just a small pillow to support your neck in its correct position. Good posture (page 148) is essential, too. If your work involves sitting at a desk, make sure your chair and desk height (page 156) are correctly adjusted to ensure a healthy posture. Pilates exercises (page 192) and learning the Alexander Technique (page 188) may also be helpful.

Keeping mobile is vitally important but load-bearing exercise, which risks over-stressing the back, should be avoided. Don't exercise with weights or run on hard ground, both of which put strain on the spine, unless your doctor says that you can. Swimming is an ideal activity, and yoga (page 196) is also recommended.

Osteoporosis

Osteoporosis, also called "brittle bone disease," is a condition in which bones gradually lose their calcium content. The bones lose density, which makes them more fragile and easily compressed. The result is an increased risk of fractured or crushed bones.

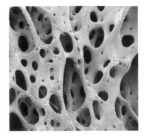

NORMAL BONE

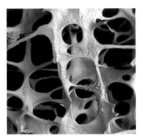

OSTEOPOROTIC BONE

The National Osteoporosis Foundation estimates that 55 percent of Americans over 50 are affected by loss of bone density. Fortunately, with proper prevention, stabilizing techniques, and medication, osteoporosis can be halted or slowed down—and in some cases reversed. The information on these pages also applies to osteopenia, an early step on the path to full-blown osteoporosis. The bones have become less dense, but the likelihood of breakage is less than with osteoporosis.

Symptoms Osteoporosis can affect most bones, but the spine, hips, ribs, and wrists are the most common sites for fractures. There are no warning symptoms, so the condition is often not diagnosed until something breaks. Over the years, repeated compression fractures of the vertebrae can lead to chronic low-back pain, loss of height, and an abnormal curvature of the upper spine, often called a "Dowager's Hump" (page 52).

What causes loss of bone density? Bone is laid down early in life, but bone-building stops around the age of 25 and it stays at the same density until about 35. Thereafter, about 0.4 percent of bone density is lost each year as part of the normal aging process. This happens because bone is a living, dynamic structure in which calcium is constantly borrowed from bones to maintain levels of calcium in the blood, then returned to build new bone. Osteoporosis results when the rate at which calcium is taken from bone is greater than the rate at which it is returned.

Prevention Throughout life eating the right diet and getting enough exercise and sunshine can prevent and slow loss of bone density. The diet should include calcium, found in dairy products, calcium-enriched cereals and orange juice, and vitamin D, which helps the body to absorb calcium. Vitamin D is also found in dairy products (most milk is fortified with it) as well as other fortified foods and oily fish. Keep in mind that most vitamin D in the majority of people is made in the

OSTEOPOROSIS CLOSE UP Modern scanning techniques reveal osteoporosis. In bone affected by osteoporosis, the proportion of bone in the mesh-like structure is considerably reduced. For an accurate diagnosis of bone density in cases of suspected osteoporosis, a DXA (dual-energy X-ray absorptiometry) scan is usually used.

skin, where its production is triggered by sunlight. So even with a good diet, you're at risk of vitamin D deficiency if you don't get at least 15 minutes' exposure a day for six months a year. The Food and Nutrition Board of the Institute of Medicine recommends the following daily intakes of the following bone-building nutrients:

- **Calcium** 800mg for children 1–10 years of age; 1,200 mg 11–25 years; 1,000 mg over 25 years, including women on hormone therapy (HT); 1,500 mg for postmenopausal women not on HT.
- **Vitamin D** 400 IU for infants under 12 months; 600 IU for children and adults under 71 years; 800 IU for those 72 years and over. Keep in mind that long-term excess of vitamin D intake can lead to elevated levels of calcium in blood and urine, that can cause kidney stones. So stay within the Food and Nutrition Board's recommendations.

Exercise is another vital element in your bone-strengthening armory. To help prevent bone loss, your bones need to experience a force generated by moving the weight of your body against the pull of gravity and the pull of working muscles. How much force your bones need depends on their current strength and density—plus whether or not you have any of the additional risk factors for the condition, such as not getting enough exercise, being thin, or having a family history of the condition.

You haven't got much control over gravity and, unless you are already very thin, there are good reasons in terms of your general health to avoid putting on weight. So the only way to put additional bone-building force on our bones is through exercise of the right kind. Any exercise that makes you bear more weight is beneficial. Walking, lifting hand weights, even just climbing the stairs

Why Exercise Builds Bone Strength ▸▸

The most likely reason why exercise—particularly weight-bearing exercise—builds bone strength is due to the action of special bone-building cells, known as osteoblasts, that form when the muscles and the bones to which they are attached are placed under pressure. The osteoblasts help the bones to adapt to the pressure and become denser and stronger.

can all help you build bone. Pilates exercises (page 192) and yoga (page 196) can also be of benefit. Swimming and cycling do not cause you to bear weight, so these activities do not greatly improve bone density. If you already have bone loss, you should avoid doing sit-ups; these have been known to cause fractures in people with osteoporosis.

Research has shown that it is more effective to do a variety of brief, regular exercises, such as three 20-minute sessions each week, rather than one long stint. Exercise regularly, because bone takes time to change. The exercises on the following pages can help increase bone density by as much as 4 percent over a year.

Should You Use Hormone Therapy? ▸▸

Taking a combination of the hormones estrogen and progestin after menopause has been shown to prevent bone loss and increase bone density. But because it also increases the risk of heart attack, stroke, and blood clots, and is associated with some types of cancer, hormone therapy is no longer advised for long-term use. Instead, it is used for only a short period to relieve particularly difficult menopausal symptoms. If you're considering it, check with your gynecologist.

Get your own program Since an exercise program depends largely upon your own bones and their condition, ask your doctor to refer you to a physical therapist to develop a program specifically designed to suit your needs.

Figuring out what's wrong The suspicion that you have reduced bone-density often only arises after you start to experience back pain or you suffer a fracture from a minor injury. In this case, your physician is likely to recommend a bone-mineral density (BMD) test—a non-invasive out-patient procedure that shows if your bones have become weakened. A DXA (dual-energy X-ray absorptiometry) scan is used. The results are compared with those of a young adult of the same sex and ethnicity and given a "T" score. Osteoporosis is defined as a bone density T-score of -2.5; osteopenia is a T-score of -1 to -2.5. Testing is advised for groups at special risk, including: people over 65; those who are thin; those who have rheumatoid arthritis or other chronic inflammatory conditions; those who have a diet low in vitamin D or calcium; and those who have not exercised regularly over many years.

Fixing the problem A range of drugs can be used to treat osteoporosis. As with all drugs, these medicines also have side effects. (For more information, see *Drug Treatment*, page 204.)

- **Antiresorptive agents** Reduce the rate at which calcium is removed from bones.
- **Selective estrogen receptor modulators (SERMS)** Mimic the bone-building action of estrogen.
- **Calcitonin** Prevents bone loss in postmenopausal women and in those with osteoporosis.
- **Teriparatide and Denosumab** For short-term use and for those at high risk of multiple fractures.

Take a Balanced Approach ▸▸

If you have osteoporosis, improving your balance is vital, because doing so reduces the risk you'll fall and break a bone. One tip: Go barefoot whenever you can. The increased contact bare feet have with the floor will help you stay balanced and upright.

THE STORK
Test and improve your balance by holding the stork position on alternate legs—but stand by a table or chair for security. Hold for as long as you can and try to build up to balancing for 60 seconds.

Exercises for Spine Strength ▸

Before doing these exercises, be sure to read the cautions on page 10.

Adapted arrow
This exercise strengthens your back muscles by making them pull on the bones of your spine.

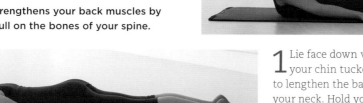

1 Lie face down with your chin tucked in to lengthen the back of your neck. Hold your hands palms down by your sides.

2 Looking down at the floor, lift your head and shoulders up. Hold for 30 seconds and lower. Repeat five times.

Alternate arm and leg stretch
This exercise has similar benefits as the adapted arrow, but with an increased pull on the whole spine.

Lie as for the adapted arrow, but with your arms forward and palms facing one another. Lift your opposite arm and leg up from the floor, but don't let your back arch. Hold for 30 seconds. Repeat with your other arm and leg, then repeat the sequence five times.

Swimming
This exercise not only helps increase bone density but it also reduces the risk of developing shoulder problems.

Lie as for the adapted arrow and bring one arm forward and one leg up. Swing the forward arm to the side and back in an arc, as you bring the other arm forward in a similar arc. Repeat five times, then lift your other leg and repeat the arm movements. Repeat the sequence five times.

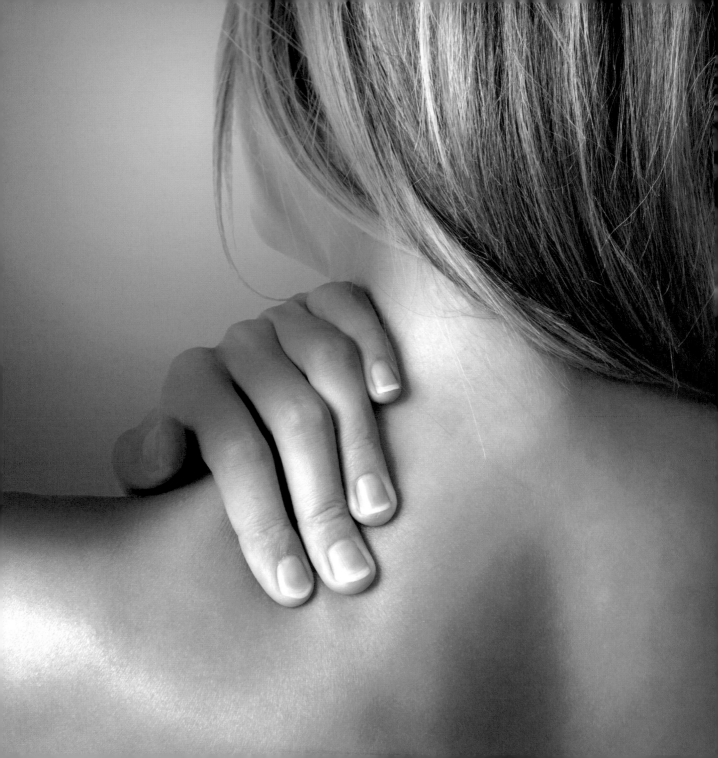

Chapter 3

Neck and Shoulders

The spine extends through the neck to the base of the skull and is closely linked to the structures that form the shoulders. Many back problems, including whiplash injuries, tension- or posture-related muscle stiffness, as well as specific disorders such as cervical spondylosis (osteoarthritis of the neck vertebrae) are primarily felt in these areas. At the end of the chapter you'll find suggestions for exercises to help you deal with the most common problems.

Shouldering the Weight

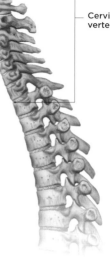

Cervical vertebrae

Our upper backs, necks, and shoulders handle quite a load every day. Tasks like carrying groceries, bending over a kitchen counter, or sitting at a desk for long periods all stress the muscles at the top of our spine. What's more, the neck has to constantly carry the weight of our head—between 10 and 13 pounds (4.5–5.9 kg), roughly the weight of a bowling ball.

The shoulder-neck connection The upper back is a complex structure, and problems in one part often lead to problems in another. For example, the muscles of the neck run down to the shoulder blade (scapula), which in turn is part of the complex shoulder girdle (page 15). Injury to any part is likely to have consequences further down the line.

If you have sustained damage to the rotator cuff—the group of muscles and tendons that keep the ball and socket joint of the shoulder in place—you will probably hunch your shoulders to protect the area and may eventually end up with a stiff neck as well. The nerves in this part of the body are also closely interconnected. A disk or facet joint problem in the neck (cervical) region of the spine may therefore bring about pain in the shoulder if the nerves are affected.

Your cervical vertebrae There are seven vertebrae that make up the cervical spine, which is far more mobile than the thoracic and lumbar regions. This mobility gives us the freedom of movement we need to move our neck and head freely.

The first two vertebrae, the atlas and the axis, differ from the others in that they are designed specifically to allow your neck to rotate in many directions, including looking to the side. Special ligaments between these vertebrae allow maximum

KNOW THE AREA
The cervical spine consists of the first seven vertebrae of the spine. They differ in structure from those of the lower spine to allow a greater range of movement.

rotation between the two bones. Though the cervical spine is very flexible, it is also at risk of injury from sudden movements, such as whiplash-type injuries (see *Accidents and injuries*, page 29).

A delicate area As well as supporting the head, the cervical vertebrae have another job. Of all the vertebrae in the spine, only these have openings for the arteries to take blood to the brain as well as space for the spinal canal carrying the spinal cord. This means that great care has to be taken if you have any sort of manipulation in this area. Whether it's done by a beauty shop operator as she washes your hair over a sink or by a chiropractor making some small adjustment, there is a risk of causing a stroke by interrupting the blood supply to the brain.

Practitioners of manipulation therapies including osteopathy, chiropractic, and physical therapy all receive training for assessing patients likely to be at risk of a stroke.

WHAT'S GOING ON?
Whether a nagging ache
or a sudden sharp pain,
trouble in the neck and
shoulders demands medical
assessment.

When To Call the Doctor ▸▸

It's a relief to know that neck pain is rarely a sign of anything life-
threatening. But there are a few symptoms that should set alarm
bells ringing. Harvard Medical School advises contacting a medical
professional right away if the pain is so severe you cannot sit still,
or if it is accompanied by any of these symptoms:

Symptom	Possible cause
Fever, headache, and neck stiffness together	Meningitis
Pain traveling down one arm, especially if the arm or hand is weak, numb, or tingling	Herniated cervical disk pressing on a nerve
Loss of bowel or bladder control	Pressure on the spinal cord
Persistent swellings in the neck	Infection or tumor
Chest pain or pressure	A heart attack or inflamed heart muscle

Neck Strain and Sprain

Although most neck problems are not serious, that is little consolation when you can't move yours more than an inch either way. Two out of three people will develop neck pain at some time in their lives. Generally, a minor strain of the ligaments, tendons, or muscles in the neck will heal in a few days or weeks. But sometimes you'll need a bit of expert help.

Symptoms When you injure the soft tissues (ligaments, tendons, and muscles) in your neck, you may not always feel the pain where you expect. It may be localized in the middle or in one side of your neck or spread to the shoulder or upper chest, the center, back, or side of your head, behind your eye, or even to your ear. It may feel like stiffness, radiating pain, a burning sensation, muscle spasm, or headache.

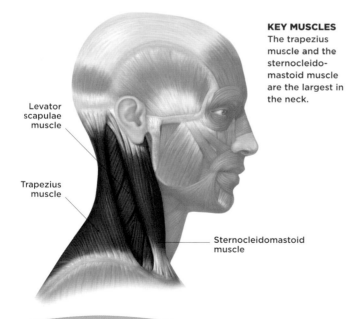

KEY MUSCLES
The trapezius muscle and the sternocleido-mastoid muscle are the largest in the neck.

Levator scapulae muscle

Trapezius muscle

Sternocleidomastoid muscle

What causes neck strain? If you're susceptible, a sudden movement—as commonplace as brushing your hair or as obvious as a whiplash injury (see page 29)—can bring on neck problems, possibly by disturbing a facet joint (page 17) in one of your vertebrae. When this happens, the surrounding muscles knot into a spasm to protect the area: it feels as if your neck is "locked" and unable to move.

The main muscles involved are those at the back and sides of the neck (see illustration, left), but the small muscles that run from vertebra to vertebra may also go into spasm (see *Muscle Up*, page 18). As long as the muscles are contracted in a spasm, they cannot receive sufficient oxygen and this makes the pain and stiffness worse.

Advancing age and pregnancy increase the risk of this type of neck pain because, in these circumstances, the ligaments surrounding the cervical vertebrae tend to loosen, and their ability to stabilize the neck is reduced.

If the nature of your job means your neck stays in one position for long periods of time—for example, driving or sitting at a desk or checkout counter—you are also more likely to develop problems.

According to the University of Maryland Medical Center, muscle strain or tension caused by everyday activities is among the commonest causes of neck pain. The major triggers are:

- Bending over a desk for hours.
- Poor posture while watching TV or reading.
- Placing your computer screen too high or too low.
- Sleeping in an uncomfortable position.
- Twisting and turning the neck in a jarring manner while exercising.

Prevention There's a lot you can do to reduce your chances of soft-tissue neck pain. Here are some tips:

Do
- Take frequent breaks if you drive long distances or work long hours at your computer.
- Adjust your desk, chair, and computer so the monitor is facing you directly at eye level.
- Stretch frequently if you work at a desk.

Don't
- Tuck the phone between your ear and shoulder. If you use the phone a lot and need to keep your hands free—say, for typing—get a headset.
- Sleep on your stomach. Lying in this position puts stress on your neck.
- Have a pillow that is too firm or too high. Choose one that supports the natural curve of your neck.

Fixing the problem When we're in pain we instinctively protect the damaged area by avoiding normal activities and movement. But this can make things worse because lack of movement can increase stiffness and weaken the neck muscles. They then tire more easily and become more susceptible to further strain.

Over-the-counter painkillers (page 204) can relieve pain and stiffness enough to give you some movement. An ice pack or heat pad may also be of benefit (see *Help Yourself!*, page 214). Ask your physician if physical therapy (page

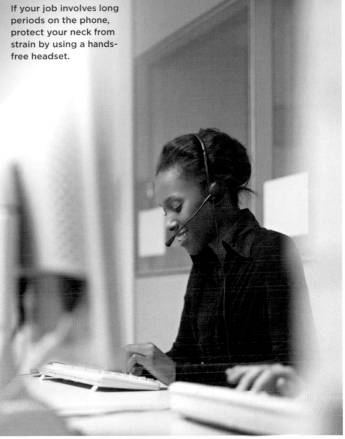

PHONE SENSE
If your job involves long periods on the phone, protect your neck from strain by using a hands-free headset.

178) or treatment by an osteopath (page 182) or chiropractor (page 184) might be helpful. If you are prone to neck problems, regular sessions of a posture-improving therapy such as Alexander Technique (page 188) or Pilates (page 192) may help to prevent a recurrence, as well. If your physician agrees and the pain allows, try the exercises on page 96. They may reduce pain and stiffness.

Stress Headaches

Chances are you wouldn't dream of blaming neck and jaw muscles for a blinding headache. But they could very well be the problem. As the muscles in both areas come under stress, they go into spasm, creating what doctors refer to as a tension headache.

Where you experience the pain depends on which muscles are affected. If the focus of discomfort is at the base of the skull, the problem is probably in the trapezius muscle (see *Key Muscles*, page 76). When there's pressure at the temple, the likely culprits are the muscles that move the jaw.

Because the neck muscles are close together and pain can be referred from one area to another, it's not always easy to tell which one is causing the trouble. Gentle pressure on each from a medical professional should help locate the problem zone.

Symptoms The kind of headaches that are caused by stress or tension—whether physical or psychological—usually cause a dull rather than throbbing pain. The ache is not specific to one area, though it may be worse in the scalp, temples, or the back of the neck. Sometimes it can feel as if you have a tight band or vise around your head.

What causes stress headaches? It's no surprise that repetitive actions—or continuous inaction—can spark problems. Any activity during which you hold your head in one position for a long time without moving can cause a headache: while you're operating a computer or keyboard, for example, doing fine work with the hands, or using a microscope. Sleeping in a cold room or with your neck in an unnatural position may be a trigger.

The causes can be emotional or psychological too. This is because our muscles contract in response to stress, depression, anger, or anxiety.

According to the U.S. National Institutes of Health, "The pain may occur as an isolated event, constantly, or daily. Pain may last for 30 minutes to 7 days. It may be triggered by or get worse with stress, fatigue, noise, or glare."

Figuring out what's wrong Always visit your doctor if you have persistent headaches—mainly to rule out a serious cause. He or she will usually be able to diagnose a stress headache from your description of the symptoms and the fact that your head and neck muscles may be tender to the touch.

Prevention If you know what triggers your headaches, you can usually take steps to avoid those actions or situations. Keep a "headache diary" and note down:

- The day and time the pain began.
- What you ate and drank in the previous 24 hours.
- When you went to bed, how long you slept, and when you woke up.
- What was going on in your life immediately before the pain started.
- How long the headache lasted.
- What made it stop.

Fixing the problem If you get a headache every day you sit at a desk for three hours, try breaking up your desk time with short stretch-and-move breaks. In fact, any time you find yourself sitting in one place for several hours, get up, stretch, and walk around a bit.

If you suspect that tension in your neck muscles arising out of psychological stress is at the root of your headaches, try to reduce the amount of strain in your life. That may mean you need to organize your day differently in order to:

- Build in relaxation time.
- Get more sleep.
- Schedule more exercise.

It's well worth trying out a few specific relaxation techniques to help you unwind (page 162). And learn good posture (page 148). According to the Mayo Clinic, good posture can help keep your head and neck muscles from tensing up by placing less strain on your soft tissues and bones.

While painkillers can be useful, you should not depend on them too heavily as regular overuse of any of these medications—particularly those that contain caffeine—can cause "rebound headaches," headaches that occur as a consequence of stopping the medication. Your doctor may suggest you try a muscle relaxant. And some antidepressants, used at very low doses, are helpful in preventing pain.

If your headaches are chronic, combining drug treatment with relaxation or stress-management training or complementary therapies such as acupuncture (page 198) may provide better relief. Try the exercises that start on page 96 and the five-minute relaxation technique on page 162.

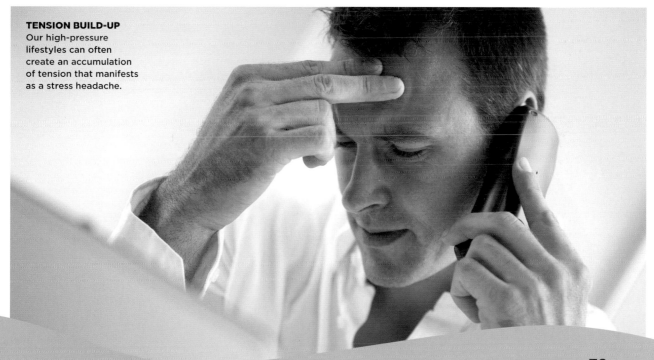

TENSION BUILD-UP
Our high-pressure lifestyles can often create an accumulation of tension that manifests as a stress headache.

Wry Neck

You will certainly know if you've had the temporarily disabling condition called wry neck, known medically as torticollis. The word literally means "twisted neck" and the condition makes you look as if somebody has taken your head and wrenched it to one side: your skull is turned one way, while your chin points in the opposite direction.

Symptoms You can go to bed feeling just fine and wake up in the morning hardly able to straighten your head and neck. As well as looking lopsided, you may also experience headache, head tremors, or neck pain. Your neck muscles will feel stiff and tender and one shoulder may be raised. Call your physician at once if you also have difficulty breathing or swallowing or believe you may have suffered a neck injury.

What causes wry neck? The cause is usually soft-tissue damage or irritation. Common triggers include exposure of the neck muscles to cold—for example, by sleeping in a drafty room—sitting or sleeping in an unusual position without proper neck support or with too many pillows, poor posture in front of a computer screen, or carrying a heavy, unbalanced load.

More rarely, wry neck can be caused by a throat or upper respiratory tract infection, which produces inflammation that can trigger spasm in the muscles of the neck. Occasionally, the root cause is an abnormality or injury of the neck vertebrae.

Some prescribed antipsychotic medications (also known as major tranquilizers), which are sometimes prescribed for those with schizophrenia, and certain recreational drugs, such as ketamine, cocaine, and amphetamines, can bring on acute dystonia, the medical term for a lack of normal muscle control. This, in turn, can result in acute torticollis.

A tendency to wry neck can run in families—when it is known as spasmodic torticollis—and usually starts with muscle spasms in middle age. Without treatment, the condition can become permanent. Babies can be born with wry neck if their head is in the wrong position in the womb or if the muscles or blood supply to the neck are damaged.

Figuring out what's wrong Your physician will probably be able to make a diagnosis by taking a history and examining you. To rule out more serious causes of your problem, he or she may send you for further tests like an X-ray or electromyogram, which picks up electrical activity to test muscle function.

Fixing the problem The good news is that torticollis usually passes within a day or two, though you may still have some symptoms after a week or more. Applying heat may ease the stiffness, and massage and manipulation may help (page 186). You could also try a soft neck collar.

It may sound impossible, but try to keep your neck moving as normally as possible. Just do not drive if you have a restricted range of neck movement as there is a risk that your range of vision will be impaired.

Rest if the pain is intolerable, but then exercise your neck as soon as you can; try not to let it stiffen up completely. Gently move your head in each direction every few hours and gradually increase your range of movement. Don't worry that you will cause damage to your neck by moving it—you won't. (See page 98 for exercise suggestions.)

Painkillers such as acetominophen or NSAIDs may be helpful (page 204). Or your doctor may prescribe something stronger such as a muscle relaxant or a drug used to treat muscle spasm—orally or by injection. According to the National Institutes of Health, injections of Botox (botulinum toxin) can temporarily relieve torticollis, but repeat injections every three months are usually needed if the problem becomes chronic. In a few cases surgery may become necessary.

In children who are born with torticollis, the aim is to stretch their shortened neck muscles; treatment is usually successful, if started early.

Cervical Nerve Root Problems

The nerves branching off the spinal cord in the neck and elsewhere are well protected. But injuries can still occur, and when they do, inflammation of the nerve root (the spot where a nerve branches off from the spinal cord) can cause severe pain in your neck and shoulders—and elsewhere. Nerve root problems in the mid and lower back are discussed on page 116.

Symptoms In many cases, damage to the nerve roots that branch from the spinal cord in the neck region causes, in addition to pain in the neck itself, pain, numbness, or tingling in the arms (brachialgia) or upper body. Obviously, if you notice such symptoms, you need to seek expert help promptly.

What causes cervical nerve root problems? The cause of this kind of problem may be a minor and temporary inflammation of the tissues surrounding the spot where the nerve slips between the vertebrae. This is popularly called a pinched or trapped nerve, known by doctors as cervical

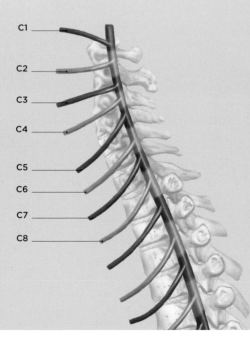

C1
C2
C3
C4
C5
C6
C7
C8

Know Your Cervical Nerves ▶▶

There are eight cervical nerves in the neck that transmit sensations such as pain, heat, and cold from the arms and upper body to the brain. Each also carries instructions from the brain to the muscles.

Nerve	Area it controls
C1 and C2	Head
C3 and C4	Diaphragm
C5	Upper body muscles, such as the deltoids on the shoulders, and the biceps on the arm, which allow flexion of the elbow and rotation of the forearm
C6	Wrist muscles and the biceps
C7	Triceps, the large muscles on the back of the arm that control elbow straightening
C8	Hands

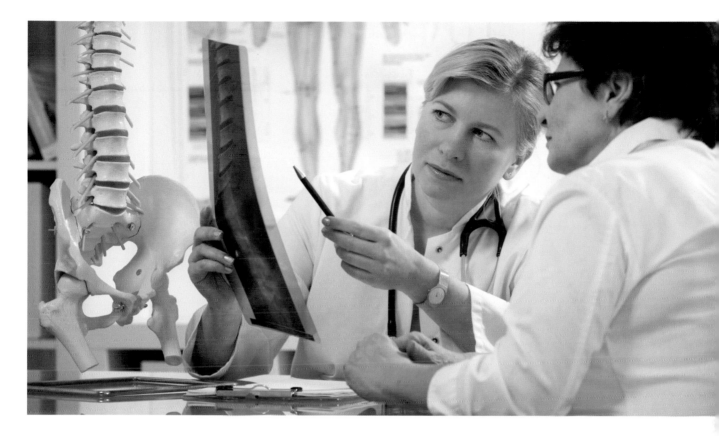

radiculopathy. Because pairs of nerves leave the spinal cord through gaps between the vertebrae, they can be easily compressed by injuries to a facet joint or to an intervertebral disk.

Various other conditions can cause a pinched nerve. One is spinal stenosis (page 116). Another is osteoarthritis (page 58), which often occurs with spinal stenosis and is an almost inevitable part of the aging process. In some people, small spur-like deposits of calcium, the mineral from which bone is formed, develop on and around the vertebrae. When these bony spurs, known as osteophytes, put pressure on the spinal cord and nerve roots, the pain can be excruciating. But the website of the American Academy of Orthopaedic Surgeons points out, "if MRI scans were performed on everybody age 50 and over, nearly half of the scans would show worn disks and pinched nerves that do not cause painful symptoms. It is not known why some patients have symptoms and others do not."

One is spinal stenosis (page 116). Another is osteoarthritis (page 58)

UNDERSTANDING YOUR CONDITION

If you have symptoms of nerve root trouble, you're likely to be given an X-ray or scan to discover what's going on.

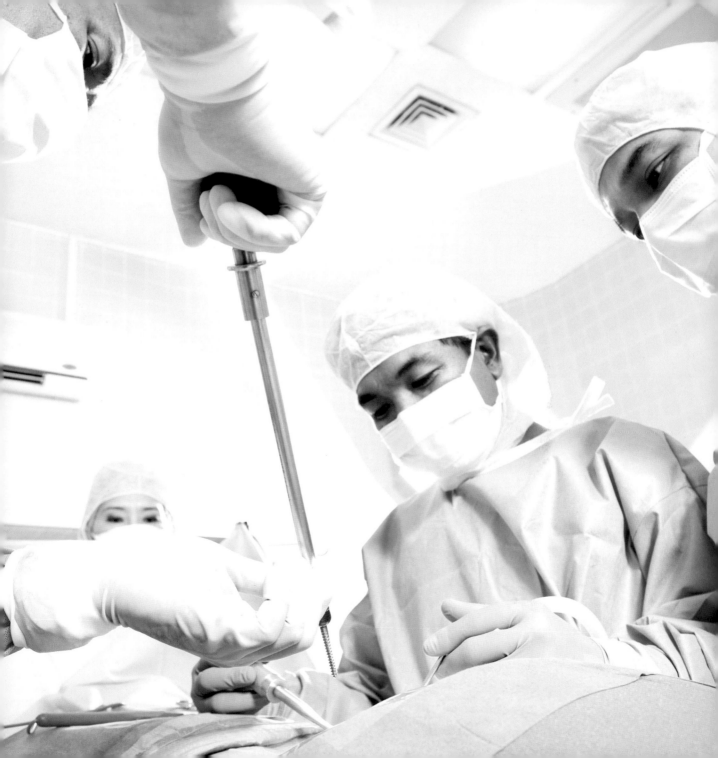

Prevention There are no specific measures you can take to prevent nerve root problems in the neck. Keep your neck flexible and strong by practicing the exercises starting on page 96 and follow the advice on posture and avoiding strain given in Chapter 5.

Figuring out what's wrong As well as asking you about your symptoms, your doctor will assess your range of movements, and may well arrange for you to have X-rays, or CT or MRI scans (see *An Expert Assessment*, page 42) to view the bones and soft-tissues in your neck.

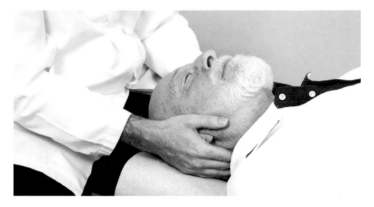

Fixing the problem Most people with nerve root irritation as a result of temporary inflammation get better without treatment. In some, the pain disappears within days or weeks, while others take longer. It is wise to avoid vigorous exercise or heavy lifting if you have nerve inflammation. And a collar or neck brace may provide short-term relief (see *Help Yourself!*, page 214).

■ **Medication** Where pain is a main symptom, painkillers and nonsteroidal anti-inflammatory drugs (NSAIDs) are often the only treatment required. In some cases, stronger pain relief medication such as codeine or tramadol may be prescribed. Muscle relaxants such as diazepam are also effective for some people. Corticosteroids administered by mouth or by injection to block nerve signals in the affected area may be given using spinal imaging to ensure the needle finds its target. (For more information, see *Drug Treatment*, page 204.)

THE SURGICAL ROUTE
Modern surgical techniques have improved the outlook for many people with nerve root irritation. But this is still an option that needs to be considered carefully.

■ **Heat and cold** Many neck problems can be alleviated by the application of heat or cold (see *Help Yourself!*, page 214).

■ **Physical therapy** Your physician may refer you to a physical therapist for therapies such as traction on the head, other forms of gentle manipulation or exercises, and possibly ultrasound treatment (see page 178).

■ **Other therapies** Osteopathy (page 182) and chiropractic (page 184) may be helpful but should only be considered on medical advice after you've had an MRI scan. Acupuncture (page 198), shiatsu (page 200), and TENS (page 202) may relieve symptoms in some cases. Ask your physician first.

■ **Surgery** If disk pain lasts more than a few weeks, gets progressively worse, or causes problems with mobility, surgery may be an option. Often a surgeon can remove just the protruding portion of the disk. But if the whole disk needs to be removed, the vertebrae may have to be fused together with a bone graft and perhaps a metal plate to provide stability. This is not an option to be undertaken lightly. The insertion of an artificial disk is also possible. (See also *Surgery*, page 210.)

TAKE IT GENTLY
Neck manipulation can be helpful, but it should be undertaken only on medical advice by a properly qualified practitioner.

Thoracic Outlet Syndrome

A complex and controversial problem, thoracic outlet syndrome (TOS) is hard to diagnose because it causes a variety of symptoms, many of which can also be caused by other, unrelated, conditions. As a result, some doctors doubt that any non-specific form of the condition exists.

The thoracic outlet consists of three passageways running beneath the shoulder from the base of the neck toward the armpit. The passageways are fairly small, and can become even smaller as a result of injury, or repetitive actions and a lifestyle that distorts the normal shape and tension of muscles or the alignment of bones. If this happens, the structures passing through them can become compressed or irritated. These structures include the blood vessels and the nerves that supply the arm, hand, and shoulder. Compressed or irritated nerves and blood vessels in this area are thought to affect between 3 and 80 of every 1,000 people.

Symptoms TOS symptoms depend on whether the nerves or blood vessels are being compressed. Since they both supply the arm and hand as well as the shoulder, signs and symptoms can occur some distance from the site of the problem.

There are two well-recognized types of TOS—neurogenic TOS, in which nerves are compressed, and vascular TOS, in which blood vessels are compressed. A third type, non-specific TOS, is more controversial and is not accepted as a distinct condition by some experts. In this form of TOS, the symptoms are clearly present, but the process by which these have developed cannot be demonstrated by tests.

Quick Relief ▸▸

To relieve the pain caused by TOS quickly, raise the hand of your affected limb and rest it palm down on your head, keeping your upper arm level with your shoulder. This will help open up the thoracic outlet and relieve any compression.

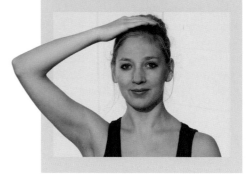

Neurogenic TOS symptoms include:

- Numbness and tingling in the neck and shoulder.
- Pain in the arm and hand.
- Pins and needles in the forearm and palm.
- Weakness and cramps of hand muscles.

Vascular TOS symptoms include:

- Deep pain in the neck and shoulder, often worse at night.
- Throbbing in the area above the collar bone.
- Bluish hands.

- Arm pain and swelling, with a weak pulse.
- Tiny black spots on the fingers.

Non-specific TOS symptoms include:

- A mixture of neurogenic and vascular symptoms because some nerves and some blood vessels may be compressed at the same time.

What causes TOS? The main cause of TOS is poor posture (page 148), as when the shoulders droop, the head is held forward and the chest is sunken—all of which tend to reduce the size of the thoracic outlet. Repetitive actions—such as typing at a computer or repeatedly lifting something above your head—also play their part in causing inflammation of the tissues and therefore narrowing of the thoracic outlet.

TOS affects women about nine times more than men, partly as a result of differences in the shape of the chest wall, and partly because large or pendulous and unsupported breasts or perhaps the posture sometimes associated with them, can make the thoracic outlet smaller.

Prevention The avoidance of repetitive actions that involve moving your arm over your head is an important part of prevention, as is the way that you hold your neck. If such movements and positions play an important part in your work, ask an occupational therapist to advise you about best workplace practice, or ask a physical therapist to show you stretching exercises that might help.

Figuring out what's wrong First, your physician is likely to put you through a series of provocative maneuvers—that is, you will be asked to adopt certain positions or make certain movements to see whether symptoms get better or worse. X-rays may be taken to check for any bone damage and find out if there is an extra cervical rib. An MRI or a CT scan may be used to reveal any soft-tissue problems. Between them, such tests can also help to rule out other problems, such as a tumor, that may be responsible for the symptoms. In some cases, an EMG (electromyography) study may be performed to evaluate nerve damage, while a Doppler blood flow study (an imaging technique that uses sound waves) may be done to check the health of the blood vessels.

An Extra Rib ▸▸

Around one in every 200 of us has an anatomical defect known as a cervical rib, which grows out of the seventh cervical vertebra above the first rib; 70 percent of people with a cervical rib have one on both sides of their body.

About 10 percent of people with a cervical rib develop TOS. But the rib itself is often not the culprit. Instead a band of fibrous tissue, invisible to an X-ray, causes the compression. If TOS becomes severe, the cervical rib can be surgically removed.

Fixing the problem Physical therapy (page 178) is the mainstay of treatment, using ultrasound, mobilizations, a specially tailored exercise and stretching program, and postural correction. Alexander Technique (page 188) can help improve posture. Osteopathy (page 182) and chiropractic (page 184) can also be effective for some people. Your physician is likely to prescribe muscle relaxants and NSAIDs (page 204) for pain relief. TENS (page 202) can also help to ease discomfort.

Unless the cause of TOS is a cervical rib or overlarge breasts, surgery is not a first line of treatment, as there is a risk of complications. In fact, it is rarely recommended until other treatments have been tried without significant success.

Shoulder Damage

Millions of Americans visit their doctor every year for shoulder injuries, often caused by repetitive movements during sports such as tennis or swimming, or by everyday activities such as carrying groceries, cleaning, or gardening.

The shoulder is one of the most complex joints in the body. According to the National Institute of Arthritis and Musculoskeletal and Skin Diseases, the shoulder is easily injured because the ball of the upper arm bone (humerus) is larger than the shoulder socket that holds it. The shoulder joint has been compared to a golf ball and tee. The shallow "cup" would permit the "ball" to slip off if the joint were not given added support by the surrounding soft tissues, namely the ligaments and the muscles surrounding the shoulder that make up the structure known as the rotator cuff. In addition, the three short ligaments that protect the joint

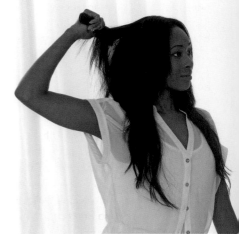

IT'S MY SHOULDER
Shoulder damage can cause pain when you lift your arm to comb your hair.

are rather inefficient and unstable. As a result, the joint's stability relies to a great extent on its short, protective rotator cuff muscles, which are easily damaged (see *Rotator Cuff Problems,* page 90).

Symptoms Shoulder pain from strain can be a dull background ache or a sharp pain that severely restricts your movement. Sometimes the pain extends right down to the wrist. It can often waken you from sleep and stretching your arm overhead is particularly troublesome. You may also experience arm weakness. Neck problems can also cause pain over the shoulder blade or in the upper outer arm (see *Know Your Cervical Nerves,* page 82).

What causes shoulder pain? Most shoulder problems are caused by overuse, poor posture, or injury and inflammation of the soft tissues—muscles, tendons, ligaments, and fascia. Other

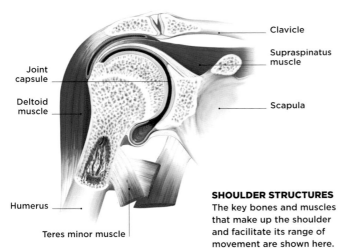

Clavicle

Supraspinatus muscle

Joint capsule

Deltoid muscle

Scapula

Humerus

Teres minor muscle

SHOULDER STRUCTURES
The key bones and muscles that make up the shoulder and facilitate its range of movement are shown here.

possible causes are fractures of the upper arm bone (humerus), collar bone (clavicle), shoulder blade (scapula) or—for reasons that are not fully understood—a build-up of calcium in the shoulder joints. Sometimes the tendons become inflamed because they are pinched by other parts of the shoulder joint, a condition known as impingement.

Many of these problems occur in the muscles and tendons that make up the rotator cuff (page 90). If the fluid-filled sac that protects the shoulder joint is also inflamed, this is called synovitis or capsulitis. Also, pain in the shoulder that is accompanied by a tingling sensation in that area is caused by something amiss in the neck region.

Prevention Stay mobile. This is the key message for anyone wishing to prevent shoulder problems. And it is particularly important to maintain mobility if you start to notice symptoms that may be an early sign of frozen shoulder. Moving the shoulder helps to break up scar tissue that may be building up in the joint. Try the exercises starting on page 96. Pilates (page 192) and yoga (page 196) are also good for shoulder mobility.

It is important to pay attention to good posture and to avoid strain (page 148). If you need to carry things, use a backpack or divide the weight between two bags—one in each hand. Try not to carry a single heavy bag over one shoulder.

Figuring out what's wrong It's likely your doctor will be able to identify the root of the problem by studying your movements and listening to an account of your symptoms. Where there is doubt, an ultrasound scan will show up any thickening in the soft tissues and can also detect the amount of fluid in the joint. It can also highlight damage to tendons and muscles. An MRI scan provides more detailed images. Sometimes a contrast fluid is injected into the shoulder before a scan or X-ray to highlight tears or blockages.

Fixing the problem

If possible, try to carry on with normal activities, without overstraining yourself. Over-the-counter painkillers (page 204), gentle stretching, and an ice pack or heat pack (page 214) may help alleviate your discomfort.

Your physician may refer you for physical therapy (page 178). And your therapist may, in turn, recommend exercises to carry out at home. In some cases, you may be advised to have a cortisone injection into the shoulder to relieve inflammation. Subject to your physician's advice, osteopathy (page 182) or chiropractic (page 184) may help. And some people gain relief from acupuncture (page 198) or shiatsu (page 200).

If shoulder problems persist after other treatment options have been tried, your physician may recommend that you consider surgery. Surgery can be used to manipulate the joint under anesthesia, remove loose pieces of bone or a calcium deposit, cut away the scar tissue in a frozen shoulder, or trim bone to prevent impingement. Much shoulder surgery is performed by minimally invasive "keyhole" techniques, which have a faster recovery time than conventional surgery.

Frozen Out ▸▸

You may well have heard of frozen shoulder, a painful condition that seriously restricts joint movement. Scar tissue grows inside the capsule of the shoulder joint, probably as a result of the cumulative effect of many tiny sprains. The presence of this fibrous tissue leaves less space in the joint and makes arm movements stiff and painful. The condition is more common in older people and in those who have diabetes, lung and heart disease, or rheumatoid arthritis.

Rotator Cuff Problems

If you suffer from shoulder and neck pain, it is highly possible that the rotator cuff is the source of your problem. According to the American Academy of Orthopaedic Surgeons, around two million people in the U.S. went to their doctors in 2008 because of a rotator cuff problem.

The rotator cuff is a complex arrangement of muscles and tendons that keeps the head of the upper arm bone (humerus) in place in the shoulder socket. This structure makes the shoulder joint both mobile and strong. Two fluid-filled sacs (bursae) smooth the movement between bones, muscles, and tendons and protect the rotator cuff from the bony arch of the shoulder blade (acromium).

The most common rotator cuff problems are tendinitis—inflammation of a tendon—and bursitis—inflammation of the bursal sacs that protect the shoulder. The two often go together. The supraspinatus muscle, the part of the rotator cuff closest to the top of the shoulder blade, is easily strained by unaccustomed frequent or repetitive actions (for example, painting a ceiling or pitching a baseball) or a sudden wrench or a blow. If this happens, the tendon becomes inflamed and thickened—a condition called supraspinatus tendinitis. The muscle is then liable to be chafed by nearby bones and ligaments, causing further inflammation and soreness. This additional challenge is called impingement syndrome.

Symptoms Once a rotator cuff problem has set in, any activity that involves lifting your arm, like getting dressed or reaching for something, can result in a shooting pain. When the rotator cuff muscles cannot move easily, those between the neck and the shoulder tend to overwork to compensate, leading to hunched shoulders. The area often feels tender. Lying on that side is painful and this may interfere with sleep at night.

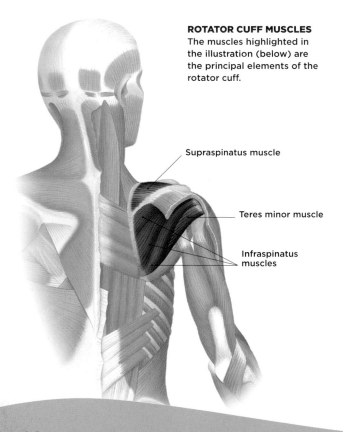

ROTATOR CUFF MUSCLES
The muscles highlighted in the illustration (below) are the principal elements of the rotator cuff.

Supraspinatus muscle

Teres minor muscle

Infraspinatus muscles

What causes rotator cuff problems? This part
of your body becomes more vulnerable to injury
as you age. Damage happens in various ways: from
sudden trauma like a fall or accident (typically when
you put your arm out to save yourself from a fall),
from continuous overuse during sports or work,
or from gradual deterioration of the muscles and
tendons due to aging.

If untreated, inflammation and impingement
can eventually lead to weakness and a tear in
the rotator cuff tendons. A tear can also happen
suddenly, due to trauma. This sounds pretty serious,
but you may not even realize that your rotator cuff
is torn, though sometimes the injury can cause
significant pain and need treatment.

Figuring out what's wrong After listening to an
account of your symptoms, your physician may
need only to make a physical examination in order
to reach a diagnosis of a rotator cuff problem. How
freely and painlessly you can move your shoulder
and arm will give pointers to where the problem
lies. If your doctor suspects impingement, he or
she may inject a small amount of anesthetic into
the space under the upper part of the shoulder

blade to see whether that relieves the pain and
restores some mobility. As it can be hard to tell by
examination whether there is a tear in the rotator
cuff, you may be sent for further tests, such as
an MRI scan (page 42).

Fixing the problem If you have tendinitis or a tear,
your physician is likely to recommend that you take
steps to alleviate the pain and inflammation with
rest, an ice pack or heat pad (page 214), and anti-
inflammatory medication (page 204).

Referral to a physical therapist (page 178)
for passive exercises (in which the
therapist gently extends the range
of movement of the joint) is usually
the next step. In addition, ultrasound
may be used as a treatment to reduce
inflammation of the soft tissues and
improve blood flow. Massage therapy
(page 186) may also be advised.
Later, your physical therapist may
recommend further gentle stretching
and strengthening exercises. (See also
Shoulder Exercises, page 100.)

If none of this works, a
corticosteroid injection into or near
the painful spot can bring relief.

For those who have been in serious
pain for many months, surgery
may be an option. This may involve
removing some bone or part of the
bursa to relieve pressure in the area.
If there is a muscle tear, the surgeon
may also carry out a repair.

A carefully planned rehabilitation
program under the supervision of a
physical therapist is essential after
shoulder surgery.

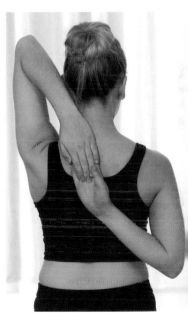

CAN YOU DO THIS?
Check out the flexibility of
your rotator cuff muscles
and tendons by trying this
simple move. If you can't
reach, regular practice may
increase flexibility.

Cervical Spondylosis

As we age, the joints in our necks show signs of wear and tear and this can lead to changes in the neck vertebrae as the body adapts to joint damage. Around 85 percent of Americans over the age of 60 experience this condition, known as cervical spondylosis, which is another term for osteoarthritis of the neck.

Symptoms The symptoms of cervical spondylosis are variable. If you have this condition, you may find that your neck has gotten stiffer over time, though the onset of symptoms can also be quite sudden. The pain may be in the neck itself, between or over the shoulder blades. If a nerve is pinched, pain and/or pins and needles can be felt from the shoulder down as far as the fingers.

You may feel numbness in your shoulders and arms and, rarely, the legs—in which case you need to seek medical advice promptly. Sometimes symptoms are worse after standing or sitting (especially in a draft), or in the morning if you slept in an awkward position, when you sneeze, cough, or laugh, or bend your neck backward.

Discomfort can be mild, or you may have pain so severe that you cannot move your head. You may have attacks of vertigo if you move your head quickly. The symptoms can be constant, or you may have flare-ups. In all cases get medical advice.

Some people in whom X-rays reveal the presence of cervical spondylosis exhibit no symptoms at all.

What causes cervical spondylosis? Age is not the only cause of wear on the bones and soft tissues of the neck. Years of regular sporting activities or doing a physical job that has placed stress on the neck can have the same effect.

According to the National Institutes of Health, there are several other risk factors for cervical spondylosis. These include being overweight and lack of exercise, a past neck injury—sometimes many years before—previous spinal surgery, a damaged intervertebral disk, and the effects of osteoporosis (page 68).

Prevention It's hard to avoid the stresses and strains of everyday life that contribute to the development of cervical spondylosis. But you can reduce their impact by paying attention to the advice on posture and lifestyle given in Chapter 5, *The Healthy Back*.

Fixing the problem It's important to keep your neck gently moving so it does not stiffen up. Over-the-counter painkillers, such as acetaminophen or nonsteroidal anti-inflammatory drugs (page 204) may help and your physician may give you something more powerful on an occasional basis for flare ups.

Your physician may recommend standard physical therapy (page 178) and perhaps complementary therapies such as osteopathy, (page 182), chiropractic (page 184), and acupuncture (page 198), which can bring relief of symptoms to some people.

Out of Alignment ▸▸

Sometimes a condition called spondylolisthesis can be a complication of cervical spondylosis. When it occurs in the neck, the condition is often termed subaxial subluxation. One of the vertebrae slips forward (if it slips backward the condition is called retrolisthesis) so it's out of line with the rest of the spine. This may happen because of progressive degeneration or due to trauma such as a motor vehicle collision. If the slippage is slight, you may not experience any symptoms. But if the misaligned vertebra presses against a nerve, the pain can be severe and you may have tingling or numbness in the arms and/or legs.

What's the treatment? The treatment for spondylolisthesis is initially the same as for cervical spondylosis. But if things do not settle down, you may need surgery. Fusion of the vertebrae around the area of slippage is an option that is often recommended, especially when there are symptoms of nerve compression. In some cases the vertebrae are moved back to the normal position prior to performing the fusion, and in others the vertebrae are fused where they are after the slip.

Neck Injuries

The thought of serious neck injury is terrifying—and rightly so.
A break (fracture) or dislocation in the cervical region of the spine can
be potentially fatal or catastrophically disabling. Thankfully, though,
few neck injuries are life-threatening.

FRACTURE AND DISLOCATION

Learning that somebody has broken or dislocated their neck is always shocking news. Fractures and dislocations usually happen in accidents, typically in an automobile crash or as a result of sports mishap. The use of seatbelts, and rule changes and protective equipment in contact sports have reduced the number of these injuries seen in emergency rooms.

Any injury in which this type of damage is even a remote possibility should be treated as an emergency and immediate medical help should be called. On no account should the person be moved unless there is an imminent, and potentially fatal threat from another source—for example, fire.

What happens? A fracture means a break in the bone, while dislocation involves displacement of the vertebrae out of their normal position. The effects can be similar. The American Academy of Orthopaedic Surgeons (AAOS) emphasizes that any injury to the vertebrae can be serious because of the risk to the spinal cord. Injury to the spinal cord can cause paralysis or death. Damage to the spinal cord in the neck can lead to paralysis.

What should be done? In all cases of serious trauma to the neck, the body is immobilized until X-rays have been taken and the person has been assessed by a doctor. Treatment depends on which of the seven cervical vertebrae are damaged and in what way.

For a minor compression fracture, a cervical brace worn for a couple of months may be adequate. A more complex or extensive fracture may need traction and surgery to stabilize the damaged area, which may entail months in a rigid cast, or a mix of these treatments.

"BURNERS" AND "STINGERS"

If you've played contact sports and suffered a burner or a stinger, you remember it. The pain shoots from the shoulder to the hand "like an electric shock or lightning bolt down the arm" as the AAOS puts it. A burner or a stinger is an injury to the nerve supply to the upper arm, either at the neck or shoulder, often following a fall onto the head—for example, following a tackle in football.

What happens? When the head is forced sideways and downward, it bends the neck and pinches the surrounding nerves. As a result, you may feel numbness or weakness in the arm and possibly a feeling of warmth.

Usually the symptoms subside quickly—within seconds or minutes—but in up to 10 percent of cases, the unpleasant sensations can last hours, days, or longer.

What should be done? You should immediately get checked by a doctor. An examination will confirm the type of injury. If the symptoms pass, you will probably need no treatment. But you may need further medical attention if you experience weakness lasting more than a few days, neck pain, symptoms in both arms, or if you have a history of recurrent stingers or burners. Having a narrow spinal canal—spinal stenosis (page 116)—may make you more prone to burners and stingers.

WHIPLASH

When your head is jerked violently and unexpectedly backward or forward—typically in a car accident or during contact sports—the resulting injury is known as whiplash. It can also be called cervical sprain (or strain) or hyperextension injury.

What happens? The pain is caused by the soft tissues (muscles, tendons, and ligaments) of the neck being forced to the very limit of their range of motion. If the ligaments are torn, there will be internal bleeding between them and the vertebrae. You may start to feel pain and experience stiffness in the neck within minutes or it make take several hours for symptoms to be felt. Further symptoms that result from whiplash may include neck spasms, dizziness, and headache.

What should be done? It's important to seek medical help as soon as possible. Modern surgical treatment with internal fixation (screws, plates, rods) has eliminated the need for cast treatment in all but the most unusual circumstances. A plastic collar may be used for a short period.

Subject to your physician's advice, painkillers (page 204) and an ice pack or heat pad (page 214) may help relieve discomfort in the early stages of the recovery process.

You can expect a full recovery within a couple of weeks, although some people have problems for longer. Research suggests that the sooner the symptoms appear after the injury, the longer they are likely to last. It also suggests that the average recovery time for a whiplash injury without any other associated symptoms is 32 days. In a study of 2,627 participants, one in eight had not recovered six months later.

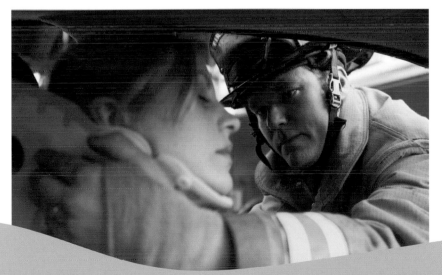

A HELPING HAND
In an accident when a neck injury is a possibility, it's vital to wait for expert emergency help. Trained paramedics have the skills and equipment to prevent further damage.

Five-Minute Warm Up ▸▸

Make sure that you choose a room that is warm, in order to help your muscles stretch and relax, and adequately aired, so that you take in sufficient oxygen to maximize muscle efficiency.

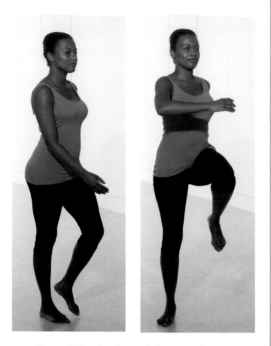

Start by walking in place while swinging your arms freely for two minutes. Then move to jogging in place, again swinging your arms, for another two minutes. Finish by marching for one minute—pulling your knees as high as possible at the same time as swinging your arms at shoulder height across and behind your body. Relax, take a few deep breaths and start your exercise routine. When you have finished, relax (page 162) for five minutes.

Neck and Shoulder Mobilizer ▸▸

This sequence is helpful in relieving conditions that cause acute and chronic neck pain (page 76). Before doing these exercises, be sure to check with your physician, and read the cautions on page 10. Remember to warm up first (left).

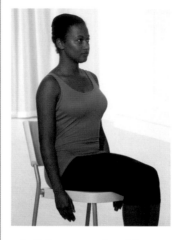 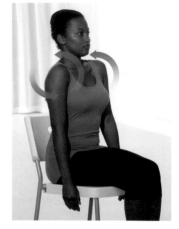

1 Sit in a neutral position (page 25) on a stool or chair and look straight in front of you, without tilting your head.

2 Using a circular motion, push your shoulders forward and up toward your earlobes and then rotate them back and down. Repeat the movement five times.

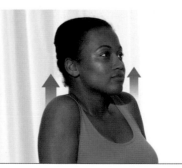

3 Raise your shoulders straight up toward your ears. Hold for 10 seconds and then allow your shoulders to drop down. Repeat five times.

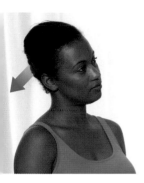

4 Look straight forward. Tilt your head down toward your right shoulder. Hold for 10 seconds, then repeat on the left side. Repeat five times, working each shoulder alternately—make sure that you do not move your shoulder toward your head.

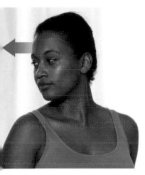

5 Turn your head to look over your right shoulder. Hold for 10 seconds and then turn to look over your left shoulder and hold for 10 seconds. Repeat five times—keep your shoulders down and relaxed and do not twist your trunk.

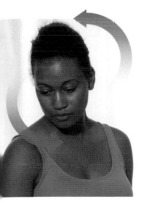

6 Rotate your head clockwise. Repeat three times and repeat in a counter-clockwise direction, keeping your shoulders relaxed and down throughout.

7 Place your right hand under your right buttock. Tilt your head to the left. Place your left hand over the right side of your head. Hold without pressure for 10 seconds and release. Repeat five times, then change hands and repeat the whole exercise.

Neck and Shoulder Exercises ▸▸

The first sequence of exercises on these pages focuses on neck mobility. They are excellent for increasing muscle strength without putting undue strain on joints which may be arthritic. You can build this exercise into your regular routine. The static stretches on the opposite page help to relieve pain and stiffness in both the neck and shoulders. They are most useful when you have a particular problem that is causing pain or loss of mobility in these areas. And the shoulder loosener (opposite) is a great way of maintaining shoulder mobility whether or not you have a current problem. Before doing any of these exercises, read the cautions on page 10.

Static neck stretches

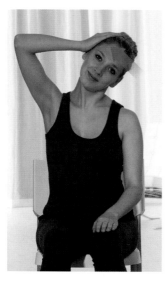 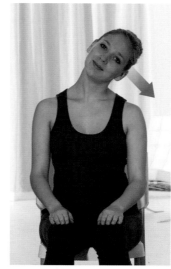 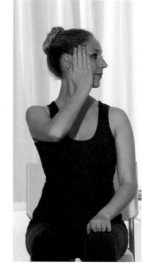 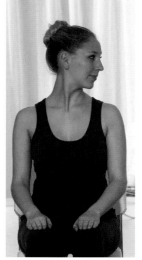

1 Sit on a stool or chair. Tilt your head down to your left shoulder as far as possible. Place your right hand over the top of the right side of your head and push your head up against your stationary hand—there must not be any movement—until your muscles start to tire.

2 Take your right hand away and then try to tilt your head further down to your left shoulder. Repeat five times, then repeat the whole sequence on the opposite side.

3 Sit on a stool or chair and turn your head to look over your left shoulder. Place your right hand against the lower right side of your face and push your head against your hand—hold until your muscles start to tire.

4 Take your hand away, and then try to look further over your left shoulder. Repeat three times, then repeat the whole sequence on the opposite side.

Wall stretch

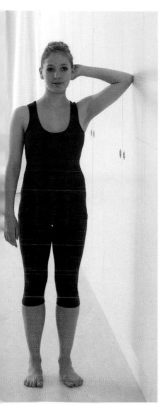

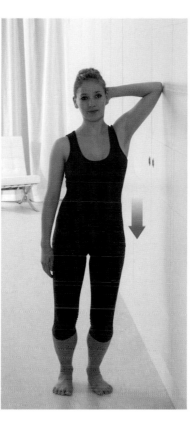

1 Stand side-on to a wall with whichever side is tight and painful next to it. Bend your elbow so that it rests against the wall, while cupping the back of your head with your hand.

2 Take a deep breath, and as you exhale bend your knees—but keep your elbow in the same position against the wall.

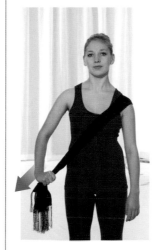

Shoulder stretch
Place a scarf or towel over the shoulder that is painful and bring both ends to meet at the opposite hip. Grasp with your hand on the same side and pull down gently. Hold for 10 seconds and repeat five times.

Shoulder loosener
Stand with your feet shoulder-width apart, your abdominal muscles tightened, and your arms by your side. Swing one arm up over your head and around like a windmill. Repeat five times. Then swing the other arm in the same way.

Shoulder Exercises ▸▸

These exercises help relieve pain and increase mobility in most conditions that affect the shoulder and general aches and pains caused by overuse and bad posture. Before doing these exercises, read the cautions on page 10.

Elephant trunk

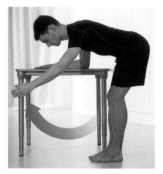 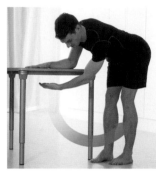

1 Stand and bend over forward, resting one hand on a chair back or table for support. Swing the other hand back and forth like an elephant's trunk 10 times.

2 Then, with your arm hanging loosely, swing the arm from side to side across the front of your body in a relaxed way 10 times.

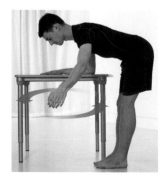

3 Finish with a circular action, first clockwise and then counter-clockwise. Do this 10 times then change sides and repeat the whole sequence.

Standing rotation

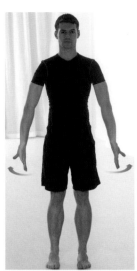

1 Stand straight, maintaining your natural spinal curves, with abdominal muscles tight, your feet shoulder-width apart, and your arms hanging down at your side. Rotate your arms so that the palms of your hand turn out to face sideways and then repeat in the other direction. Move slowly but rhythmically. Repeat five times, making sure that your shoulders stay relaxed and down and do not hunch forward.

2 Repeat Step 1 but hold your hands out to the side at shoulder height.

Hands-to-back stretch

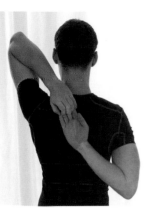

1 Stand straight with your feet shoulder-width apart and place one hand as far down your back as possible. Place the other hand on your back as far up as possible and try to interlock the fingers. Hold for a count of 10 and then change sides.

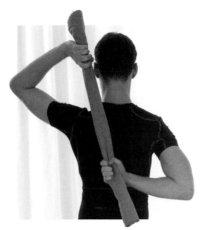

Alternative If you can't touch your fingers, hold a scarf (or belt) in the top hand and let it dangle down your back. Grasp the scarf with your lower hand as far up it as possible. Gently pull down on the scarf and then pull up with your upper hand. Repeat 10 times and then swap sides.

Pole rotation

2 Lift the pole—keeping it horizontal—over your head.

3 Bring the pole down behind you. Try not to bend your elbows or let one arm lead. Reverse the movement to bring the pole back to the starting position. Repeat 10 times. To make the exercise easier, move your hands further apart, to increase the stretch, bring them closer together.

1 Stand upright with the spine in its neutral position and your abdominal muscles tightened. Hold a pole, stick, or broom handle, at either end in front of you, horizontally across the front of your body.

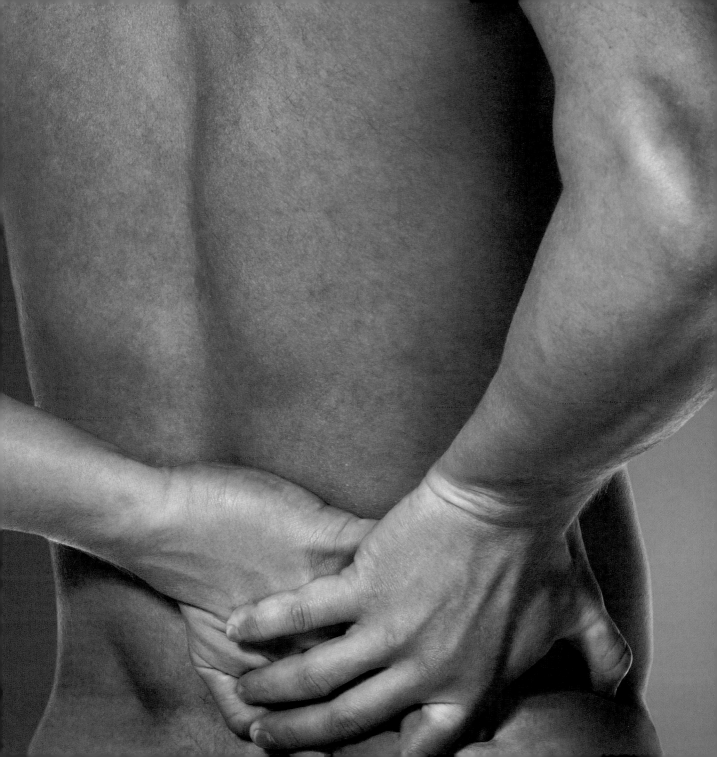

Chapter 4

Middle and Lower Back

The middle and lower back is where the majority of problems that interfere with our lives are located. In this chapter you'll find out about how the middle spine relates to the ribs, and how these structures in turn affect—and are affected by—the heart and lungs, as well as the different conditions that can affect this region of the spine. You'll also learn about the relationship between the lower spine and the pelvis and the disorders that can arise there. The chapter concludes with exercise suggestions for easing problems in this area.

Middle and Lower Back Challenges

The middle (thoracic) and lower (lumbar) back bear the weight of the upper body, which puts them under particular pressure. This makes these areas of the spine particularly vulnerable to damage and injury from both everyday movements and unusual stresses and strains.

The lumbar spine's range of movement enables you to twist. The thoracic spine has a lesser range of possible movement, but it enables you to bend forward and lean backward.

Your thoracic spine is important, too, because it moves every time you take a breath. Since your ribs are so closely linked to your spinal bones by joints and ligaments, every time you breathe in, your ribs rise; every time you breathe out, they fall.

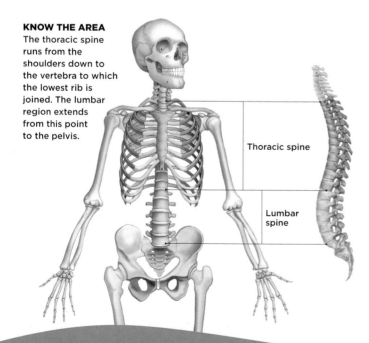

KNOW THE AREA
The thoracic spine runs from the shoulders down to the vertebra to which the lowest rib is joined. The lumbar region extends from this point to the pelvis.

Thoracic spine

Lumbar spine

What can go wrong? In this section of the book, we're going to look at what the different components of the thoracic and lumbar spine should be doing and what can go wrong when disease, injury, or other factors affect their ability to perform their usual function.

Unfortunately, there are many things that can go wrong—soft-tissue injuries (page 110), sciatica (page 118), a slipped, or "prolapsed," disk (page 116), osteoarthritis (page 58), spinal stenosis (page 116), facet joint problems (page 117), pain that has been "referred" from other parts of the body (page 36), injuries (page 122), sacroiliac joint problems (page 124), piriformis syndrome (page 128), and the special problems experienced during pregnancy (page 130). The list seems long, but there is effective treatment for most of these problems.

Tight muscles (page 114), whether in your back, hip, hamstrings (the muscles at the back of your thighs), or the deep muscles that are attached to your vertebrae are all vulnerable to strain and injury. The risk of such injury is made more likely by the sedentary lifestyle that many of us adopt, which increases the risk of losing flexibility in these key muscles (page 112).

The best way to protect your spine from injury is to pay attention to your posture (page 148) and exercise every day to maintain flexibility and keep your back healthy (page 164).

MOVE BACK TO HEALTH
Regular exercise of the right kind is the key to maintaining and restoring the health of your mid and lower back.

The Middle Back at Work

Your middle back—the thoracic region of your spine—essentially provides stability. Its range of movement is fairly limited when it comes to bending forward, bending backward, or twisting your back from side to side. But it plays a vital role every minute of your day as you breathe, and it protects your heart, lungs, and other organs in your chest from injury.

The thoracic spine consists of 12 thoracic vertebrae that play an important role in keeping your body upright. But the stability that this demands also limits how far and in what direction this area of the spine can move. The main restriction to movement is that your thoracic vertebrae have joints with your ribs and your sternum (breastbone).

The end of each rib is attached at the back to your spine. The first seven ribs are also joined to your sternum, in front. The three lower ribs are attached to the single rib above them and not directly to your sternum; the last two—called "floating" ribs—are not joined to your sternum at all, but only to the vertebrae in back.

THORACIC SPINE AND RIBS
These illustrations show the close relationship of the ribs to the spine.

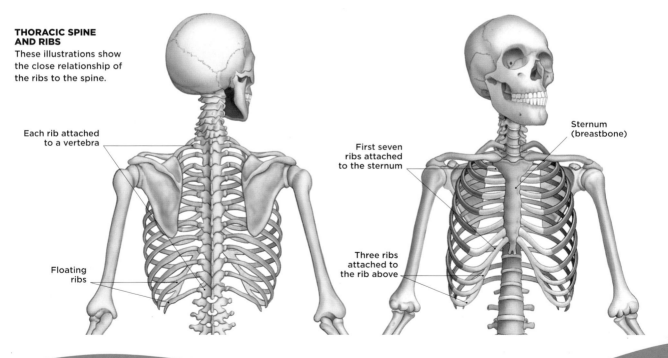

Each rib attached to a vertebra

Floating ribs

First seven ribs attached to the sternum

Sternum (breastbone)

Three ribs attached to the rib above

This means that while your lower thoracic spine is capable of an increasing range of movement, movement in its upper part is considerably limited—in fact, the range of sideways movement of the spine is only 4 degrees at the top of the thoracic region, compared with about 20 degrees in the lumbar spine.

There is a sound reason for this lack of flexibility. The thoracic spine has to be stable to protect your internal organs. But movement in some directions is necessary to allow your ribs to rise and fall when you're breathing.

What can go wrong? Injuries, such as fractures of the spine or ribs (page 120), and conditions that can affect any area of the back (see Chapter 2, starting on page 46) are the cause of some of the most serious problems that affect the middle back. But a little-known additional cause of trouble in this area is the effect of incorrect breathing.

If you breathe mainly using the muscles of your upper body, not only will your breathing be inefficient, but you will put extra strain on your thoracic spine and the muscles and ligaments that support it. The scalene muscles, which run from the cervical spine to your top two ribs, are especially at risk from this type of strain.

You are most likely to breathe in a way that may cause strain when you are under physical and emotional stress. In such circumstances you are apt to breathe faster, more shallowly, and forget to use your diaphragm to breathe efficiently. The result can be that your scalene muscles tighten up, which can cause neck pain, which in turn can affect your general posture. The converse is also true: bad posture (page 148) can lead to poor breathing technique and can therefore cause tension in your scalene muscles.

How's My Breathing? ▸▸

Check out your breathing technique by observing your abdomen while you are breathing in. Does your tummy and the area of your chest just above it move out when you breathe in? If it doesn't, you're not using your diaphragm to its full capacity while breathing and you may strain sections of your spine. The answer? Practice diaphragmatic breathing (page 136).

Learning and practicing diaphragmatic breathing so that it becomes second nature is the key to avoiding back problems caused by poor breathing technique. You can learn to become more aware of the way you breathe and how to improve it by building the diaphragmatic breathing exercise (page 136) into your regular routine. And be sure to bring attention to your breathing whenever you feel stressed.

TAKING THE AIR
From time to time make the effort to use your diaphragm fully as you breathe—your back muscles and your mind will feel more relaxed.

Low-Back Lowdown

While your middle back gives your spine stability, but only a limited range of movement, your lower back—that is, your lumbar and sacral spine and tailbone—allows your body to move in all directions. But in order to achieve this, your pelvis and related muscles must also be brought into action.

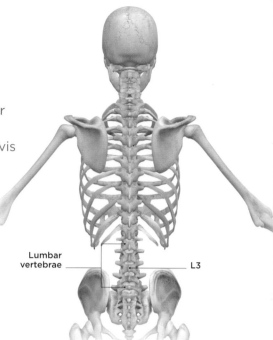

LUMBAR LOCATION
The five lumbar vertebrae take most of the strain of back movement and L3 (see *Comparing the Strain*, right) in the center of the lumbar region takes more than most.

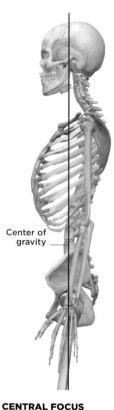

CENTRAL FOCUS
The muscles of the spine are constantly working to keep our weight evenly distributed around the center of gravity.

Your lower spine and your pelvis are inextricable linked when it comes to moving your back—which means that problems in one area can either cause or be caused by problems in the other.

Your body's center of gravity lies in front of your spine, on your chest side. That means that the muscles of your spine must work continuously to counter the pressure to bend forward and align your center of gravity more closely to your spine. In the upper and middle back, the work is done by the paraspinal muscles (page 112). These muscles do their work in the lower back, too, but they need more help to support your weight, counter torque (page 24), and, at the same time, facilitate and control twisting, leaning forward, and leaning back.

The lumbar spine is specially designed to solve these problems. It has the largest vertebrae in the spine and a natural lumbar curve (see *The neutral zone*, page 25) that provides the ideal alignment between the lumbar spine and the pelvis.

What's more there are strong muscles that run between the lumbar vertebrae and hips, such as the iliopsoas (page 19) and the quadratus lumborum (page 114). As well as providing stability, these both contribute to flexion and extension, while the paraspinals play the main role in rotation.

So what can go wrong? The most common lower back problems are caused by soft-tissue injuries (page 110) such as muscle strain and ligament damage.

It's important to realize that the strain on your lower back varies according to your posture (see opposite) and any activity that you're undertaking

Comparing the Strain ▸▸

The strains on your lumbar spine increase considerably as you move from standing upright to sitting, through slouching forward to sitting and slouching forward—in the last position strain in this area of the back is as much as twice that when you're standing upright. In the table below you can check out the comparative loads on the L3 vertebra when you are in different positions.

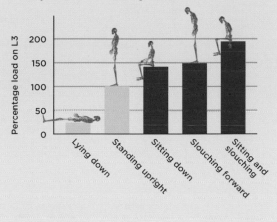

Percentage load on L3

Lying down · Standing upright · Sitting down · Slouching forward · Sitting and slouching

PROTECT YOUR LUMBAR SPINE
Working with your back in a low-stress neutral position dramatically reduces the load on your lumbar region.

such as lifting can be particularly hazardous if undertaken from a high-strain posture. What's more, if you lift something when your back is bent forward and your lumbar curve has been straightened out, especially if the weight is carried away from your body, the strain on your spine increases considerably. The result is that you're much more likely to suffer an injury.

So always lift with your back straight, your lumbar curve in the neutral zone, and the weight held close to your body (page 153). And make the middle and lower back exercises (page 134) part of your daily healthy back routine.

Soft-Tissue Injuries

Most people experience back pain at some point in their lives—85 percent of us, it's estimated—and usually it's the lower back that's involved. The reason is that this area supports most of your body's weight. Most pain is caused by soft-tissue injuries, which are believed to responsible for up to 97 percent of cases.

Two-thirds of the time you'll never know what caused a problem. Fortunately, however, most soft-tissue troubles are the result of minor strain and resolve themselves within a few weeks.

What are "soft tissues?" Basically, anything that isn't bone. That means ligaments, intervertebral disks (page 16), muscles, tendons, and connective tissue (page 18).

Any number of things can cause soft-tissue injuries in your lower back, including: poor posture, bad lifting techniques, sudden, unexpected movements—especially those that involve twisting or carrying heavy loads, such as gardening and clearing the yard. Other causes can be a sudden jolt—as you may experience in a minor car accident or a sports injury—or some external force that exacerbates the effects of an underlying disease process such as osteoarthritis (page 58).

One common reason for soft-tissue injuries is an imbalance in your muscles, in which some have become shortened and tight, and others weak and overstretched. The cause? A sedentary lifestyle.

Fast onset or slow burning? When low-back pain comes on quickly, it's said to be "acute," and you may need to take immediate action (page 38). The pain can vary widely—from a dull ache to a pain so severe you feel unable to move. But acute low-back pain usually resolves within three to six weeks and the only necessary treatment may be ice, painkillers, physical therapy (page 178), and advice from a health professional: typically, "keep moving." The days in which doctors routinely advocated days of bed rest for affected patients are long gone.

It's only if there are other signs—such as nerve pain down the leg (sciatica, page 118), numbness, bladder or bowel problems, or if the pain intensifies rather than settles—that your doctor is likely to order tests and investigate further.

"Chronic"—that is, persistent—low-back pain is classed as such if it lasts longer than six to eight weeks. The pain may be continuous, but more commonly it fluctuates between episodes of mild to moderate pain and bouts of severe pain (page 40).

To start with, you may well be treated in the same way as if you had acute low-back pain, and you're likely to be advised to keep as active as possible with the help of painkillers and NSAIDs (page 204).

If your problem persists, you may be referred to a physical therapist (page 178) who will give you an individualized exercise routine, and help you mobilize your joints. Sometimes, too, people with chronic low-back pain respond well to cognitive behavioral therapy (CBT). This aims to reduce your pain by altering the way you think and feel about it and how you behave in relation to it. For some people, osteopathy (page 182), chiropractic (page 186), acupuncture (page 198), shiatsu (page 200) or TENS (page 202) provide relief. Ask your physician's advice.

The evidence suggests that to prevent further episodes of either type of low-back pain, you need to keep active, exercise your whole body to achieve flexibility and strength—Pilates (page 192), yoga (page 196), walking, and running are ideal. Be sure to maintain good posture (page 148)—Alexander Technique (page 188) can help with this—and take care when lifting (page 152).

So what can go wrong? To look at the soft tissues of the spine, let's start from the outside and work our way in to the innermost part.

Inflamed fascia The fascia is the connective tissue that separates and encloses the different tissues in the body (see page 18). Inflammation can be a particular problem in the fascia that surrounds the muscles of the lower back. If it becomes tight, back stiffness can result. To maintain a healthy fascial network, you need to move your body regularly, within its correct range of movement, stretching tight muscles and strengthening weak ones. Damage to fascia can be treated by myofascial release techniques (page 186).

Ligaments Ligaments are strong fibrous bands (page 18) that hold your vertebrae together, allow movement at their joints, stabilize your spine, and protect your disks from untoward pressure. If a ligament is sprained or torn, the result is usually a dull, nagging pain. With incorrect spinal curves (page 52) one ligament can become overstretched and the opposing one tight. And since ligaments don't have a generous blood supply, they heal slowly—more slowly, in fact, than a fractured bone.

To avoid problems, watch your posture. If you experience ligament problems, you are likely to need to take painkillers (page 204) and have physical therapy (page 178).

KEEP YOUR SOFT TISSUES IN SHAPE
Muscles, ligaments, and tendons love to be used, so keep them in good condition with regular exercise—and boost your general health at the same time.

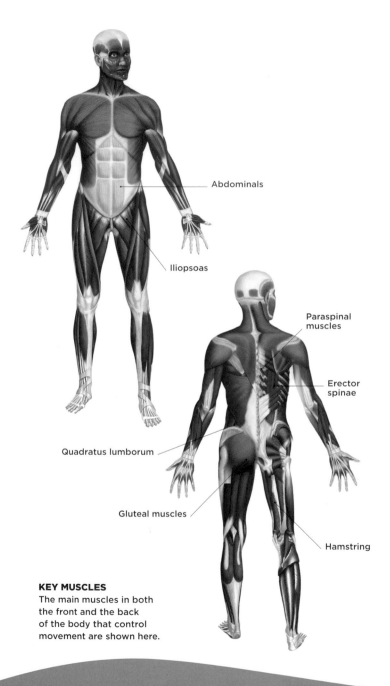

Abdominals

Iliopsoas

Paraspinal muscles

Erector spinae

Quadratus lumborum

Gluteal muscles

Hamstring

KEY MUSCLES
The main muscles in both the front and the back of the body that control movement are shown here.

Intervertebral disks These disks (page 16) are positioned between the vertebra to act as shock absorbers so they can absorb most of the pressure on the spine from walking, running, jumping, and sitting. And while some movement is vital in order for the disks to absorb moisture and remain plump, too much can cause damage and too little can result in the disks flattening and drying out.

Unfortunately, as you age the disks dry out and are less able to absorb the shocks of everyday activities. A thin disk forces the bones closer together (which is why we shrink with age), pressurizing the facet joints (page 16), and decreases the space through which the nerves pass. The result can be arthritis of the joints, pinched nerves, and slack ligaments.

To maintain good disk hydration you need adequate rest—when you lie down for an extended period, the disks plump up overnight by absorbing water from the surrounding tissues. Sitting or standing still squashes the disks, but normal movement enables them to absorb fluid and nutrients. On the other hand, overstretching—as when lifting and twisting with your back muscles— damages the disks and can cause a bulge or rupture (page 116). You need to try to find a happy medium that balances your back's need for both restorative rest and movement.

MUSCLES

Underlying most back problems are muscles that have become either too tight or too weak because of a sedentary lifestyle. A sitting position, for example, shortens some muscles, overstretches others, and weakens many. And tight, inflexible muscles put extra stress on the other muscles, ligaments, fascia, and joints. Let's take a look at the muscles involved.

Hamstrings When they're tight, these three large muscles at the back of the thigh can cause low-back pain. Many people have tight hamstrings as a result of sitting for long periods. The problem can start in school and often continues throughout life, as a result of sedentary lifestyles. When sitting, the hamstrings are inactive and shortened. Over time this becomes and feels like their "normal" state.

Shortened hamstrings cause your hips and pelvis to rotate back, flattening the lumbar curve at your lower back and causing poor posture and back problems. They also prevent your hips from flexing fully during forward bending, which in turn forces your lower back to bend beyond its normal range.

To test whether your hamstrings are tight, lie on your back on the floor, then bend both knees to right angles. Straighten and then raise one leg as far as you can. If you are only able to achieve an angle of less than 80 degrees from the floor, your hamstring is tight. So take a look at the hamstring stretches on pages 164 and 194.

Iliopsoas This abdominal muscle stretches from the lumbar vertebrae to the head of the femur (thigh bone, page 19) and helps control lower back posture. Again, it is sitting for long periods that causes problems because the iliopsoas shortens. This compresses the lumbar vertebrae, which can

Test the Tightness of Your Hip Flexors ▸▸

There are a number of variations on this test, which checks whether the iliopsoas and other muscles that flex the hip (page 18) are overly tight. If the test reveals tightness in the hip flexors, you should do regular stretching exercises (page 164) You can try this at home. Be sure to test both hips by bending each leg in turn.

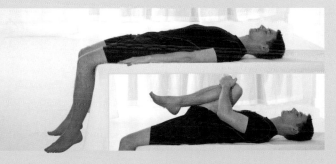

The test
Lie on your back on a table, with your lumbar spine flat and your legs dangling over the side. Pull one leg up into your chest. Check the position of your other leg.

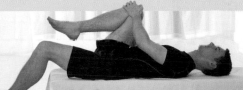

Supple flexors
If your the non-bent leg is in the same relaxed, dangling position as when you started, your hip flexors are supple.

Tight flexors
If the lower leg lifts up from the table, your hip flexors are tight.

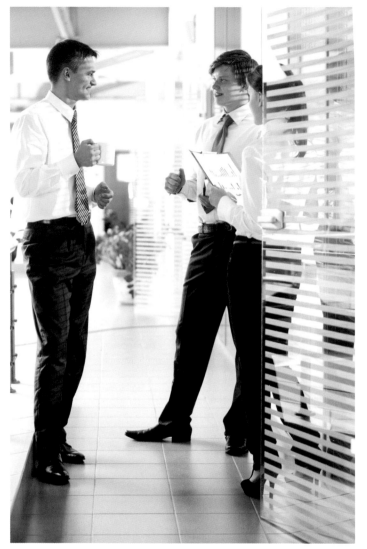

OFFICE WORK ON THE MOVE
Try to find reasons to get up from your
desk, such as meeting with your colleagues
face-to-face instead of talking on the phone.

lead to arthritic degeneration and make them susceptible to injury. It also inhibits the correct movement of the gluteal muscles (see opposite), which leads to the other back muscles having to compensate and overwork. Tight overworked back muscles equal back pain.

To avoid a tight iliopsoas, sit square in your chair (page 156)—and don't hook your feet under it. Stand and walk about frequently, strengthen your gluteal muscles (see opposite), and stretch your back and hip muscles (page 164). Test the tightness of your hip flexor muscles (see page 113) to find out if you have a problem.

The paraspinal muscles Also called the "multifidi," these are a series of deep back muscles (page 18) that lie next to the vertebrae; each one spans two to four vertebrae. Their main role is to control movement in the spine. They allow it to rotate (twist) and extend (lean backward). They also help to maintain correct posture: a neutral spine (page 25). Research shows that the paraspinals contract before you take any action in order to protect and stabilize your spine—for example, if you bend to pick up a book from the floor, your paraspinals contract fractionally before the bending movement, to prevent injury.

Many people with low-back pain have weak paraspinals that do not contract adequately before and during movement. That not only leads to less stability and support for the intervertebral joints, but underused muscles become weaker so the risk of injury increases. To work your paraspinals, try the back strengthening exercises starting on page 169.

Quadratus lumborum These are two deep-back muscles that extend from each twelfth rib down your lumbar spine and attach to the top of your pelvis (page 18). They bend your lumbar spine to the side, hike your hips up, and stabilize your lower back. Acting together, they extend your lower back and act when you breathe out forcibly—as when you cough or sneeze. They also help your diaphragm manage general breathing.

The quadratus lumborum is easily damaged by poor lifting techniques—especially when bending and twisting at the same time, such as when you load groceries from a cart into the trunk of your car. Muscle spasm or damage to the muscle fibers can cause acute, deep, back pain, making standing upright and walking difficult. The pain, often in the flank can be referred deep into the buttocks, and is usually one-sided. To keep your lifting muscles trim, check out the *Walking the dog* and *Stretch and curl* exercises on pages 170 and 171.

Abdominals The abdominal muscles, "abs," (page 18) are at the front of your spine. Rectus abdominus, the one nearest your skin, gives the "six pack" look when it is extremely well toned. The deeper abdominal muscles support the spine and control posture. Sitting, and especially slouching, shortens and weakens your abs so that the lumbar curve becomes flattened, causing stress on your vertebral joints and disks. Weak abs also fail to support the spine adequately when you bend forward or lift, which strains other muscles, joints, and ligaments, resulting in back pain. And, because your shortened weak abs overstretch your back extensors, a slouched, hunched posture can be the result. To avoid back problems from weak abs, look at the exercises on pages 170 and 194.

Erector spinae The three separate muscles that make up erector spinae (page 18) are thickest at your lumbar spine and the rim of your pelvis and thinnest at your neck. They support the back of your spine and allow you to bend backward or rotate your spine. But our sedentary lifestyles mean that they tend to be overstretched and so tire easily, giving inadequate support to the spine and a slouched posture. They can also be affected by repetitive lifting, as in manual labor, which rapidly exhausts the muscles and increases the strain on the lumbar spine, with subsequent strain on the paraspinals and quadratus lumborum, and compression of the disks and facet joints.

For exercise advice to help you avoid such problems, see pages 169–170.

Gluteal muscles The three gluteal muscles (the "glutes") are in your buttocks (page 18). Unfortunately, the glutes are inactive when you sit down, and, if not used enough, they become weak. This means that your spine extensor muscles (erector spinae, the paraspinals, and quadratus lumborum) have to work doubly hard to compensate, and you risk injuring both them and your disks.

Weak glutes can also cause hamstring pain, because your gluteus maximus muscles, the main ones, control rotation and co-ordination of your hips when walking and running. If they're weak, your hamstrings compensate and become overstretched—which is especially problematic if they're already tight—and in the worst case can cause painful tears of the muscle fibers.

Also, unfortunately, just walking and climbing stairs does not fully activate and strengthen your glutes once they've become weak. To strengthen them, try the following exercises: *Adapted arrow* (page 71), *Buttock lift* (page 168), and *Stretch and curl* (page 171). Or take up jogging, crawl swimming, or dancing.

Pressure on the Nerve Roots

A variety of conditions can cause pressure on one or more nerves as they leave your vertebral column in the middle and lower back. And, depending on the cause, the severity of symptoms, also known as "radiculopathies," can vary. Pressure on the nerve roots in the neck is discussed on page 82.

Symptoms Pressure on the nerve roots often causes what is known as "radicular pain"—that is, pain that seems to come from some distance away from the site of the original problem. This is because the nerves that emerge from your spine form the link between your brain and your outlying tissues: if they are pinched or damaged, you'll feel pain in the areas that they supply (page 21).

The symptoms of nerve root trouble in the middle and lower back can vary from back pain and numbness to nerve pain (see *Sciatica*, page 118). Bending forward or sitting tends to relieve the pain of spinal stenosis (below) because this flexed position enlarges the space available for the spinal cord or cauda equina (page 21), a bundle of nerves at the end of the cord. There may no symptoms until the condition has been present for some time. In other cases, there's an immediate onset of pain.

What causes pressure on the nerve roots?
There are a number of ways a nerve root can become compressed in this area:

Spinal stenosis A narrowing of the canal and bony openings (foramina) through which the spinal cord travels and the nerve roots emerge, spinal stenosis can cause a number of nerve root problems in the lumbar spine. The lower part of the lumbar region is more often affected than the upper part.

Spinal stenosis is usually the result of the aging process, when osteoarthritis (page 58) sets in and your disks become drier and shrink. The growth of bony projections—spurs, called osteophytes, that protrude into the canal and foramina can also contribute to nerve root problems.

Other causes of spinal stenosis are a herniated or bulging disk, inflamed facet joints, a vertebra that has slipped forward (spondylolisthesis, page 94), trauma (such as a road accident or fall from a ladder), scoliosis (page 54), bone disease, a tumor of the spine (page 50), or a congenital defect of the spine, such as a narrower than usual spinal column that has been present from birth.

Disk bulges and "slips" Unfortunately poor movement patterns, such as bending with your back rather than your legs to pick up things, can damage the innermost rings of your vertebral disks (page 16). The damage gradually spreads to the outer rings, allowing the gel-like fluid in the center to leak out. If the outermost rings are still mainly intact, the fluid causes a bulge, which can press into the central spinal canal or into the space where the nerves leave your spine, and pinch them—causing, for example, problems such as sciatica (page 118). If all the rings are damaged, and the fluid seeps out of it, the disk ruptures and "slips"—what doctors call a "prolapse" or "herniation."

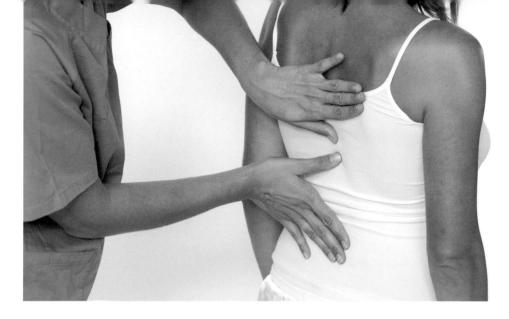

A CAREFUL ASSESSMENT
When consulting a specialist—whether a physician or physical therapist—about a nerve root problem, a thorough physical examination is likely to be the first step.

Facet joint problems These tiny joints (page 17) are located at the back of the vertebrae (page 14). They are the joints at which the upper part of each vertebra joins the lower part of the one above it, and the lower part joins the upper part of the one below. But if, for example, the lumbar spine loses stability, as a result, say, of poor lifting technique, the fibrous tissue surrounding the facet joints can thicken in an effort to regain stability and protect the area. This can not only pinch nerves as they leave the vertebral column, it can encourage the growth of bony spurs called osteophytes that will also pinch the nerves (see *Osteoarthritis*, page 58).

Figuring out what's wrong Back pain should always be investigated by your doctor. In particular, if you experience bowel and bladder incontinence, severe numbness down the legs, muscle weakness, poor balance, or paralysis, seek immediate medical attention. Following a physical examination and listening to an account of your symptoms, your physician will probably be able to make a preliminary diagnosis. An X-ray, CT scan, or MRI of the spine may confirm the precise cause. (See *An Expert Assessment*, page 42.)

Fixing the problem Many cases of nerve root inflammation get better without treatment. If this doesn't happen, the treatment options your doctor may consider include:

- **Physical therapy** This provides a personalized exercise program that usually involves stretching and strengthening exercises (page 178). Posture and movement training are also likely to be included. Massage and hot and cold packs are used to ease pain.
- **Medication** NSAIDs, painkillers, and steroid injections (page 204) may be helpful.
- **CBT (cognitive behavioral therapy)** A form of counseling that can help you understand chronic pain and cope with it better.
- **Surgery** May be an option to relieve pressure on your spinal cord and/or nerve roots (page 210).

Sciatica

People talk about sciatica as if it's a condition, but in fact it's not—it's a collection of symptoms that can involve considerable pain, often far away from the site of its cause—pain that is sometimes severe enough to incapacitate. Fortunately, there are a variety of treatments and self-help measures that can tackle the problem.

Symptoms True sciatica is pain that runs down the back of the leg and that may progress right down to your foot. Only one leg is affected. Often, the pain is described as "burning," "stinging," "numb," or "shooting." It is severe, and may preclude you from walking and taking part in normal activities. In some cases, you may also feel pain in your lower back.

What causes sciatica? Sciatica is one of the most common nerve root problems of the lower back (page 116). In fact, some 3 to 4 percent of Americans suffer from sciatica every year. It is caused by pressure on the nerve roots that emerge from the vertebral column, which then merge to form the sciatic nerve—the thickest and longest nerve in the body. The effects may also be felt in the branches of the sciatic nerve in the lower leg. Pressure can occur for any of a variety of reasons, including disk prolapse (page 116), piriformis syndrome (page 128), or spinal stenosis (page 116).

Prevention The only way to prevent sciatica is to reduce the likelihood of conditions that may cause these symptoms (see above).

Figuring out what's wrong You'll need to see your family physician if you experience the symptoms of sciatica. Try to remember what you

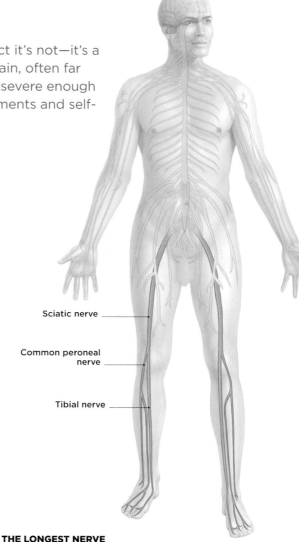

Sciatic nerve

Common peroneal nerve

Tibial nerve

THE LONGEST NERVE
The roots of the sciatic nerve emerge from the vertebral column in the lumbar region, then join together in the pelvis to run down the back of your thigh. Its branches run down the back of your calf to your foot.

were doing before the pain started, and note which positions are comfortable and which are painful so you can share the full story.

Your physician will examine you and perhaps arrange for tests based on your account of the circumstances in which the problem arose and other symptoms you may be experiencing. (See also *An Expert Assessment*, page 42.)

Fixing the problem In most cases, an attack of sciatica resolves itself within a few weeks. Your physician is likely to recommend you take painkillers (see page 204). Most spinal specialists do not advise bed rest and instead suggest continued gentle activity. Further treatment will depend on the underlying cause, but in many cases, the symptoms of sciatica resolve without additional medical intervention.

While symptoms persist, you can use a number of self-help techniques to help relieve your discomfort. Here are some dos and don'ts for the first 24 hours:

Do

- Even though the pain may be in your leg, apply an icepack to the small of your back. That's likely where the problem begins. A bag of frozen peas is ideal, but cover it with a towel because ice can burn if it is placed directly on the skin.
- If the ice is no help, press a thermal heat wrap or heating pad to the small of your back (page 214).
- Take a painkiller as advised by your doctor. Those that have an anti-inflammatory effect (page 204) are often recommended.
- If the pain is severe when resting in bed, try lying on your back with a pillow under your knees. If you turn on your side, place the pillow between your knees.

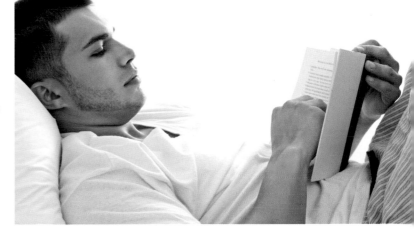

RESTING FOR RELIEF
Sometimes rest is just what your back needs. But don't stay immobile for long—it could make matters worse.

- Take note of which positions are comfortable and which are painful and let your body's natural aversion to pain dictate the position in which you should lie.
- Distract yourself with books or e-readers and try not to worry about what you should be doing instead of resting. The tension generated by worry could tighten your muscles and worsen your problem.
- Call your doctor if your symptoms show no sign of improvement in 24 hours.

Don't

- Ignore the pain: it may be a sign of damage.
- Bend, lift, twist, or carry anything.
- Let anyone unqualified manipulate your back— gentle massage that avoids the spine itself is all that anybody unqualified should attempt.

Rib Problems

When you think about your ribs, you tend to concentrate on the ones at the front of your chest. But, of course, they're connected to your spine, too, at the back. Which is why many problems that develop in your ribs affect your back as well. Unfortunately, the precise cause can be difficult to diagnose because the pain they cause can be linked to a variety of factors.

Symptoms The symptoms of rib problems are pain, either localized or over part of the chest, and pain on breathing deeply, coughing, sneezing, and laughing. Several things can be responsible, including strains, sprains, and fractures. Other conditions can also cause similar types of pain.

RIB CONNECTIONS
Each rib is attached at the back to the spine by a joint called the costovertebral joint.

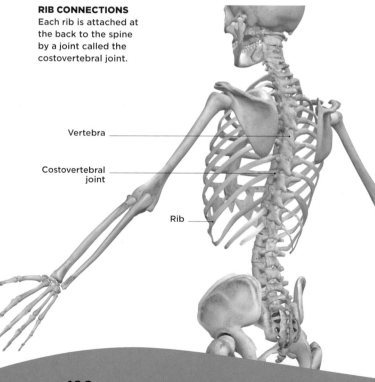

Vertebra

Costovertebral joint

Rib

What causes rib problems? Rib problems that cause back pain fall into two main groups:

Costovertebral joint strains Each rib is attached to the spine (see illustration, left), and the joint is termed the costoveterbral joint. It is supported by cartilage and ligaments. Causes of costovertebral joint strain include:

- **Muscle imbalances** Tight chest muscles and weak back muscles.
- **Working overhead** As in painting ceilings, hanging curtains, or lifting objects up and down from high shelves.
- **Poor posture** While working at a computer (page 156) or in a car (page 157).
- **Conditions** Bronchitis, asthma, or other problems that cause you to cough and sneeze a lot.
- **A poor sleeping position** Possibly caused by an unsupportive mattress or by falling asleep in an armchair.

Ligament sprains Ligaments bind and surround the costovertebral joints (above) at the spine and also where the ribs attach to the sternum (breastbone) at the front—the costochondral joints (page 106). The ligaments and cartilage surrounding these joints can be sprained—pulled or torn suddenly, especially in areas that are carrying the most load and strain—which tires the surrounding muscles. Possible causes include:

- **Chest trauma** This may be caused by a car accident or a fall. Such accidents are also often associated with rib fractures (see right).
- **Excessive movements** Including bending, lifting, arching, or twisting.
- **Sports** Especially if you're not in good shape. Contact sports such as football and ice hockey carry a particular risk.
- **Falls** These may result from an accident in the home or at work, or from participation in sports such as skiing, gymnastics, or horseback riding.
- **Carrying heavy loads** For prolonged periods.

Figuring out what's wrong First, your doctor will want to rule out a prolapsed or bulging disk in your neck or mid-back because the pain that these cause can be similar to that of a rib problem. Then your doctor will touch and manipulate the joints and ligaments involved before diagnosing the problem.

If a rib fracture (see right) is suspected, X-rays may be needed to confirm the diagnosis; if multiple rib problems are suspected, a CT or MRI scan may also be necessary.

Certain conditions can mimic rib pain and need to be eliminated by your physician. Pleurisy (inflammation of the lining of the lungs), chronic bronchitis, pneumonia, tuberculosis, lung cancer, and angina are among them.

Fixing the problem In the case of both costovertebral joint strains and ligament sprains, the first port of call is a pain-relieving medication, such as an NSAID or acetaminophen (page 204). Next comes physical therapy (page 178), with exercises,

Rib Fractures ▸▸

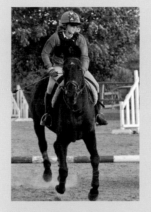

PROTECT YOUR RIBS
It makes sense to help yourself to avoid rib injuries by wearing the appropriate protective gear when doing high-risk sports.

Simple rib fractures Can be caused by chest trauma, as in a motor vehicle accident, but older people sometimes fracture a rib as a result of a simple fall—especially if their bones are weakened by osteoporosis (page 68). Younger people tend to experience fractures as a result of sporting activities, such as football or horseback riding—as well, of course, as a result of accidents. Young children are less likely to fracture a rib because their ribs are more elastic and so are resistant to impact injuries.

Fracture damage Usually, when a rib is fractured, damage occurs either at the point of impact or near to where it joins the spine at the back—structurally speaking, this is its weakest area. In itself, a simple rib fracture is not dangerous, and since you can't fix a plaster cast to a rib the only treatment is painkilling medication (page 204) while the injury heals. But it can be serious if an internal organ—most commonly the lung—is damaged by the broken bone, in which case surgery may be needed. That's why any time you suspect you've broken a rib, see your doctor immediately.

ultrasound, and massage (page 186)—both of which aim to reduce inflammation, increase joint mobility, and relax any possible muscle spasm. A physical therapist will also advise you about how to treat an underlying cause by correcting your posture (page 148) and any muscular imbalances. You'll also learn how to lift, carry, and breathe correctly.

Breaks and Bruises

Injuries to the spine's vertebrae are usually minor, but, in some cases they can be extremely serious—around 250,000 Americans have a spinal cord problem caused directly by a vertebral injury. The results can be life-changing, as well as life-threatening. Nevertheless, injuries of this type are relatively rare, and most can be treated successfully.

What causes breaks and bruises? Generally, vertebral injuries occur as a result of a fall, a car accident, a contact sport injury, or violence. Half of all of them occur in the thoracic and lumbar spine (especially in men) while women are more vulnerable than men in the tailbone area (see below). The sacrum (page 14) can also be affected by such accidents.

Many injuries just cause painful bruising, but more serious ones may cause a fracture. There are three main types: a vertebral compression fracture, in which the front of the vertebra breaks and collapses, while the back part stays stable; an axial burst, in which back wall of the body of the vertebra breaks; an extension fracture, in which two vertebrae are pulled apart; and, more rarely, a rotation fracture, in which one vertebra is moved sideways away from the vertebra above or below it. It's the rotation fracture that is most likely to cause serious spinal cord injuries.

Figuring out what's wrong If there is any suspicion that a vertebrae has been injured, especially if you have overwhelming back pain, have lost consciousness for a while, or have no feeling in the lower or other parts of your body—don't change your position or allow anyone else to move you. Instead, stay put and immediately call—or, better yet, ask someone else to call—911 or your local emergency services. The paramedics will carefully transport you to a local hospital where doctors will examine you, ask questions about your health, and about how you got injured. A neurological examination is likely to follow, with your reflexes being tested as well as your ability to sense and move your limbs. Finally, X-rays and CT and MRI scans are likely.

Fixing the problem Severe injuries are likely to require surgery (page 210), but lesser ones are treated with painkilling and anti-inflammatory medications (page 204) and physical therapy (page 178), which will include individually tailored exercises and a rehabilitation plan. Bracing is commonly needed for several weeks following a spinal fracture. Ask your physician before trying therapies such as osteopathy (page 182) or chiropractic (page 184) during rehabilitation.

TAILBONE PROBLEMS

Your tailbone (coccyx) consists of the lowest three to five vertebrae in your spine (page 14)—the variation is because often some of them are fused. The individual vertebrae vary from person to person in both shape and size, though what they have in common is that they are solid, because the spinal

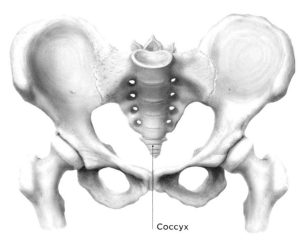

Coccyx

Fixing the problem Treatment is by means of painkilling medications (page 204), the application of ice to reduce bruising, and advice not to sit for long periods—if you have to, using a cushion with a hole in its center may help to relieve pressure.

Normally, tailbone problems clear up within a few weeks. But in some cases, tailbone pain can persist for a long time (coccydynia), and an MRI scan may be needed to get to the root of the problem. Painkilling injections and, rarely, surgery may be advised for persistent coccydinia.

cord does not run through them. The structure is particularly exposed in women, whose wider hips offer less protection than in men—indeed, the tailbone can occasionally sustain damage during childbirth. Otherwise, most tailbone injuries are the result of a fall onto it, a blow, as in contact sports, friction, as in bicycling, or, less commonly, the growth of bony spurs called osteophytes (page 58), injuries to other parts of the spine, and infections.

The good news is that because the spinal cord does not pass through the tailbone, there is no risk of damage to the spinal cord as a result of a tailbone injury.

Symptoms The symptoms vary, but are likely to include pain, tenderness, and bruising, discomfort when sitting, pain when moving your bowels, and, in women, discomfort during sex.

Figuring out what's wrong Diagnosis of tailbone injuries is initially by means of a rectal examination, to discover any damage to the coccygeal bones; an X-ray may be taken for confirmation.

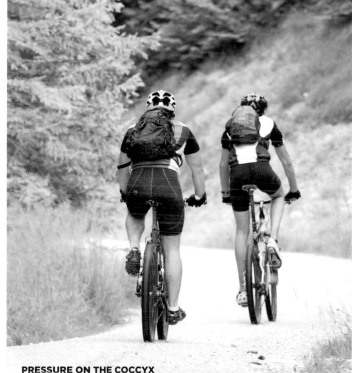

PRESSURE ON THE COCCYX
Cycling for long periods is a leading cause of tailbone injury. A careful choice of bicycle saddle may help to reduce the risk.

Sacroiliac Joint Problems

The sacroiliac joints, which are located on either side of the spine in the lower back, transmit most of the forces that the body has to absorb during daily life to the legs and feet. Unfortunately, problems with this part of the back are fairly common.

The sacroiliac, or "SI" joints as they are sometimes called, are an integral part of the pelvis. They literally join the pelvis' iliac bones to the sacrum—a section of five fused vertebrae at the end of your spine. Fortunately, given their key location, these joints are protected by a number of strong ligaments that help keep everything stable. These two tiny, L-shaped joints are estimated to be responsible for more than 20 percent of low-back pain. Injuries, muscle imbalances, whole-body conditions like osteoarthritis that affect many joints, and the hormonal changes that come with pregnancy can all predispose you to having a problem with one or both of them.

Symptoms When something goes wrong with the sacroiliac joint, the main symptom is pain—usually in the lower back and the back of the hips, but sometimes in the thigh and groin. The pain is often worse when standing and walking, but becomes better when you lie down. Sometimes there is pain in one buttock, especially while turning over in bed, and, during the day, you may find it more comfortable to put your weight on one buttock rather than the other. Some people also find that they are more prone to fall over, partly because of a feeling that their hips are unstable. There may also be mild sciatica (page 118).

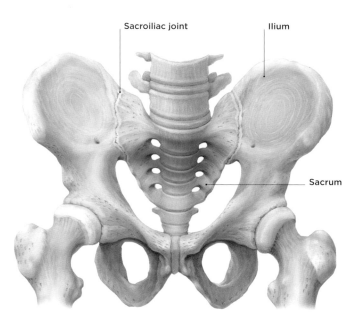

Sacroiliac joint   Ilium

Sacrum

SACROILIAC JOINTS
These joints on either side of the spine join the sacrum to the pelvis. They have a very limited capacity for movement but can become inflamed and painful as a result of injury or disease.

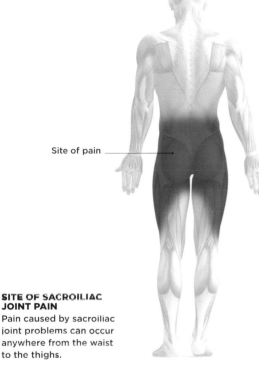

Site of pain

SITE OF SACROILIAC JOINT PAIN
Pain caused by sacroiliac joint problems can occur anywhere from the waist to the thighs.

As Common as a Cold? ➤

It's estimated that over your lifetime you have a 95 percent chance of experiencing low-back pain—which puts its incidence on a par with having a common cold. And research tells us that between 13 and, possibly, 30 percent of all back pain is caused by sacroiliac joint problems.

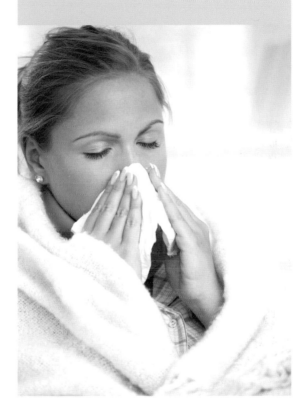

What causes sacroiliac joint problems?

Problems can arise when the cartilage that lines the joints becomes worn. This can occur for a variety of reasons. Injury is a common cause, especially when the onset of pain is sudden, but osteoarthritis (page 58) is often the main culprit.

Other conditions that can affect the sacroiliac region include rheumatoid arthritis (page 62); ankylosing spondylitis (page 66); pregnancy—because the hormones the body produces during this time relax the ligaments, so increasing the range of movement; the skin disease psoriasis; gout (the collection of uric acid crystals in joints); an abnormal gait—sometimes as a result of one leg being longer than another, or in other cases simply the result of pain in other joints.

A nerve root injury (page 116) can cause pain that is similar to sacroiliac joint pain, but this is likely to have a different cause.

Prevention The sacroiliac joints are not significantly involved in movement or posture, so there's only a limited amount you can do to keep them problem free. But it's always sensible to take care of the general health of your back, including being posture-aware (see page 148) and

maintaining a healthy weight (page 158). Check out the prevention advice in the sections of the book dealing with the possible causes of SI pain.

Figuring out what's wrong Your physician will first want to find out if your pain is due to an underlying medical condition such as those noted above. If blood tests, X-rays, and scans show that no other conditions are responsible, he or she is likely to check for any inequality in the length of your

A KEY SYMPTOM
In many cases the location of the pain or the movement that provokes pain can be a key indicator of the cause of the trouble.

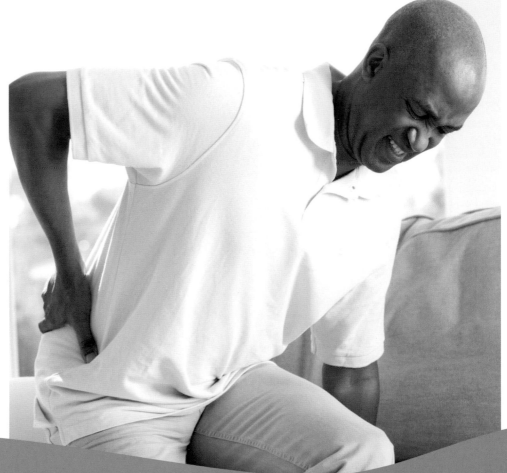

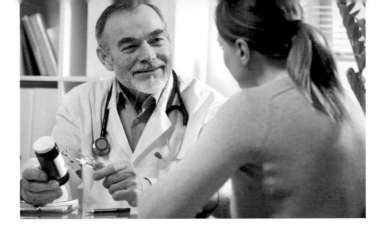

legs, and check the tilt of your pelvis. Your SI joints will probably be assessed by pressing on them—though often you are the best person to indicate precisely where the pain is by pressing your thumb at its source and showing your doctor.

Then there may be the somewhat dauntingly named "pain provocation tests," in which your physician will place you in set positions and apply pressure to your legs to judge your responses. In one such test, known as the "Gaenslen's test," you pull one knee up to your chest, while your doctor pushes your other leg downward. In another, the "FABER test," also known as the "Patrick test," you place your knee up toward your chest while your same leg is crossed over your other one; pressure is then applied to your knee.

The trouble is that research shows that none of these tests are to be considered absolutely reliable when it comes to diagnosing SI joint problems. Accurately figuring out what's going on is mainly down to your doctor's experience and instinct.

If your doctor suspects an SI problem, he or she may suggest anesthetic injections into the joint. If these relieve your symptoms, this will confirm the diagnosis of an SI problem.

Fixing the problem A lot can be done to solve your problem, but the approach to your treatment will vary depending on whether the problem is acute—in other words, of sudden onset, as after an accident or sports injury; chronic, developing slowly and lasting for longer than three months; or due to an underlying disease process. If the latter is the cause, treatment is likely to concentrate on the underlying process.

But in all cases, your doctor will likely prescribe physical therapy (page 178), which may involve stretching exercises (page 140), massage, hot and cold treatments, and ultrasound. Braces and belts to compress the buttocks may also be suggested, and if a leg-length discrepancy is the root cause, special exercises and a special insole may be advised. A physical therapist will devise a personalized treatment plan.

Medication, too, is important. NSAIDs, acetaminophen, and muscle relaxants (page 204) can relieve pain and give the joints time to improve naturally with the help of physical therapy. A variety of complementary therapies may also be of benefit (see *What Might Work*, page 176). But ask your physician's advice first.

When the problem has become chronic, injections of anesthetic and corticosteroid drugs may also be advised. As a last resort, surgery to fuse the joints may be considered if the condition is longstanding and no other options are available.

What can I do to get better? The most important thing is to focus on rehabilitation once you are over the immediate problem. Your physical therapist will recommend a detailed exercise program that you can put into practice several times a week. And be sure to avoid any activities that you have been told might make your problem worse.

TAKING THE MEDICINE
Medication is a key treatment for sacroiliac joint problems. Relief of pain can enable you to resume everyday activities.

Piriformis Syndrome

This condition mimics the symptoms of other conditions, and some experts feel that it should bear the name of those conditions. Other experts disagree and feel that it should bear the name that it does here. The good news is that symptoms can be successfully treated by a range of measures.

The piriformis is a small, flat, pyramid-shaped muscle that originates in the front of the sacral vertebrae (page 14) and runs through the pelvis to the top of the femur. Its function is to rotate the hip or, in certain positions, to turn it outward.

Normally, the sciatic nerve (page 118), which runs from the spine right down to the toes, passes beneath the muscle. But in about 15 to 20 percent of people it runs through rather than under the piriformis, and this makes it more likely that the sciatic nerve can be compressed by muscle spasm or injury (which is thought to trigger the syndrome in about 50 percent of cases). Yet the nerve can become compressed even if it does not run through the muscle.

Some estimates suggest that women are six times more likely to suffer from piriformis syndrome than men—although there is no accepted explanation of why this should be.

Symptoms Essentially, the symptoms of piriformis syndrome are the same as those of sciatica (page 92): an aching, sometimes sharp pain running down the course of the sciatic nerve in the back of the leg, particularly in the buttock area. There may also be pain in the lower back. In addition, a proportion of sufferers from piriformis syndrome notice a reduced range of movement at the hip joint.

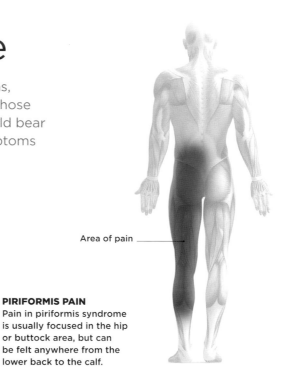

Area of pain

PIRIFORMIS PAIN
Pain in piriformis syndrome is usually focused in the hip or buttock area, but can be felt anywhere from the lower back to the calf.

What causes piriformis syndrome? Injury, trauma, and muscle spasms that result from bad posture (page 148) can all be responsible. And if your sciatic nerve passes through, rather than underneath, the piriformis you are more likely to have these symptoms.

Prevention Adopting and maintaining good posture (page 148) is the only preventive measure, although this may not be effective if the problem is triggered by an injury to the muscle or an anatomical abnormality.

Figuring out what's wrong Since it's debatable whether the condition exists or not, diagnosis is problematic and cannot be supported by tests.

Nevertheless, your physician is likely to ask for X-rays and possibly magnetic resonance imaging (MRI) to rule out any other conditions. But a scan is not always conclusive and diagnosis often relies on your symptoms and the absence of any other identifiable cause for them.

Fixing the problem The mainstay of treatment is physical therapy (page 178), in which an individual exercise program that likely includes the exercise shown on this page will be prescribed. Ultrasound (page 180) may also provide pain relief. Rest from any activities that may have triggered an underlying injury or spasm, anti-inflammatory medication (page 204), and massage therapy (page 186) have also been shown to be helpful. Osteopathy (page 182) and chiropractic (page 184) may also be effective for some people.

Does It Exist? ▸

The jury is still out. A diagnosis of piriformis syndrome has been controversial ever since the condition was first described in 1928. The main problem is diagnostic tests can suggest that you have the condition but not conclusively confirm that you have it. Nevertheless, the argument—though not the evidence—for piriformis syndrome, convinces many doctors that it is a very real problem.

Surgery to rearrange the piriformis muscle fibers so they don't impinge on the sciatic nerve can be effective, but is usually only considered when other treatment options have proved ineffective.

Exercise for Piriformis Syndrome ▸

The piriformis stretch
Lie on your back with your knees bent at right angles. If the pain is on the right side, place your right ankle just above your left knee (if the pain is on your left, substitute "right" for "left" in these instructions). Be sure to read the cautions on page 10 before you start.

Lift your right knee up toward your chest. Using your left hand, pull your right knee over to your left side. Using your right hand, grasp just above your right ankle and pull it up towards your right shoulder. Hold the position for 10 seconds, but be careful not to overstretch. As you get used to the exercise gradually build up to holding for 60 seconds. Repeat several times a day.

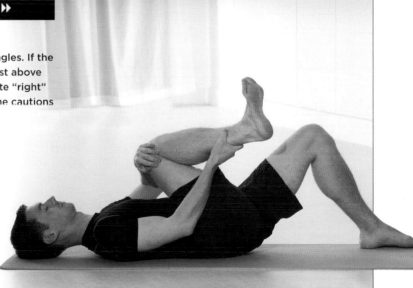

If You're Pregnant

Between 50 and 75 percent of women get back pain—particularly low back pain—during pregnancy. That's not surprising, considering the weight you gain, changes in your posture and gait, and the effects of relaxin—a hormone that loosens up your muscles and ligaments in preparation for the birth. But there are things you can do to prevent or ease your discomfort.

There are two main types of back pain that are common during pregnancy. One occurs when your muscles, ligaments, disks, or joints are strained by poor posture, bad lifting techniques, weak, tight, imbalanced muscles, and ligament strains—all of which are almost an occupational hazard of pregnancy. The second type is what's called "pelvic girdle pain" (PGP), which affects the pelvic joints.

Less commonly, back pain during pregnancy can be a sign of an underlying problem. So consult your physician if your pain is constant or intensifies or becomes unremitting—this is especially important if you also have a vaginal discharge. Remember, too, that a low, dull backache can signal the start of labor—so call for expert help immediately if you experience this.

Posture-related back pain Your posture and the pressure placed on your postural muscles changes a lot during pregnancy as you adapt to your changing weight. For example, the weight of your growing baby and increased bust size bring forward your center of gravity. So to maintain your balance, your back muscles have to work harder. As a result, your pelvis tends to tilt forward, exaggerating your lumbar curve (see also *Hyperlordosis*, page 56). Carrying extra weight and the change in your center of gravity place stress on the back muscles, joints, and disks. And your stretched stomach muscles may not be able to adequately support your spine.

What you can do There a number of things you can do that might prevent posture-related back pain in pregnancy.

Do
- Maintain good posture (page 148) and regularly practice pelvic tilts (page 134).
- Lift and bend correctly (page 152).
- Exercise to strengthen your abdominal, back, and pelvic muscles.

BALANCING THE BUMP
Back pain in pregnancy can often be the result of the change in your center of gravity that is the result of the increasing size of the baby in your belly.

Sciatica in Pregnancy »

It used to be thought that sciatica (page 116) during pregnancy is caused by your baby pressing on your spinal nerves, but the current view is that pregnant women get sciatica for the same reason as anyone else. So forget old wives' tales, you don't have to put up with the discomfort. Consult your doctor if sciatica is troubling you.

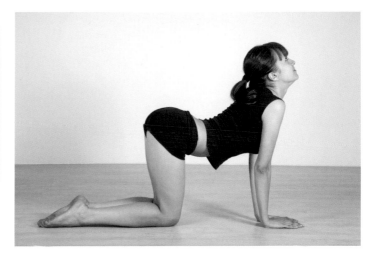

- Get a good night's sleep, especially as your pregnancy advances. Sleep on your side with one or both knees bent. Try a support pillow under your stomach, too, and between your knees—or invest in a full-length body pillow.
- Wear the right shoes: flat or low-heeled shoes that support the arches of your feet. High heels increase your lumbar curve even further than naturally occurs in pregnancy.
- Avoid standing still or staying in the same position for too long: doing so overstretches your ligaments and muscles.
- Get a maternity support belt or wear maternity panties with a low, supportive waistband.
- Use heat, cold, and massage. Use heat on your lower back to relax tense muscles. Try a warm bath, a shower, or heating pad—or try alternate ice and heat packs—to relax your muscles.
- Get onto your hands and knees in the cat position (see right) as this takes the weight of your baby off your back and can ease back pain. With your back roughly flat, breathe in and then, as you breathe out, squeeze your pelvic floor muscles. (See also *Build Support*, page 132.)
- **Don't** Sit with your legs crossed, which can throw your pelvic joints out of alignment.

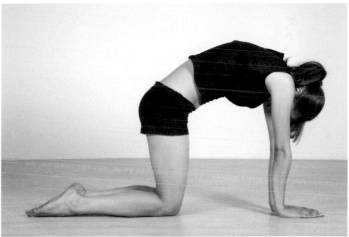

STRETCH LIKE A CAT
This is a simple and safe yoga-based exercise for back pain in pregnancy. Kneel on hands and knees, raise your head, and allow your back to sag. Then drop your head and arch your back. Repeat three times.

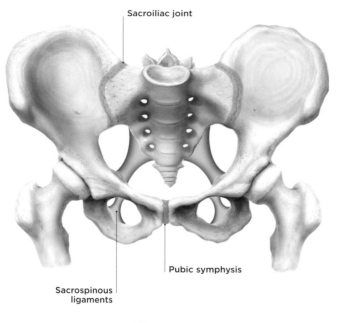

Sacroiliac joint

Pubic symphysis

Sacrospinous
ligaments

YOUR FLEXIBLE PELVIS
The normally rigid structure of the pelvis
becomes more flexible during pregnancy
as the action of the hormone relaxin softens
the ligaments in the pelvic area.

Build Support ▸▸

Kegel exercises strengthen the pelvic floor
muscles that support the uterus, the intestines,
and bladder. Strong pelvic floor muscles help
to stabilize the pelvis, so easing low-back and
pelvic girdle pain. They also help to prevent stress
incontinence, which can be a problem after giving
birth. Here's how you do them:

- Identify your pelvic floor muscles by trying to
  stop the flow of urine when you urinate. If you
  can do this, you are using them.

- Practice tightening these muscles when you
  are not urinating. Hold them tightened for 10
  seconds, then relax. Repeat five times in a row.
  Do the whole sequence five times each day.

- Try to label certain activities in your mind as
  "Kegel time." For example, when waiting for
  a bus or train, as a passenger in a car, when
  standing at a checkout, or when watching TV.

Pelvic girdle pain (PGP) Also called "symphysis
pubis disfunction" (SPD), this is common during
pregnancy and in the postnatal period, owing to the
effects of the hormone relaxin.

Normally there is little movement in the sacroiliac
joints (page 124) during everyday activities in which
the muscles "lock" the pelvis in a stable unit. But in
some pregnant women the pelvis does not lock, so
that the sides of the joints rub against each other,
causing swelling, inflammation, and pain.

The symptoms are pain in the front of your
lower abdomen over your pubic symphysis—that
is, the joint at the front of the body that links the

two sides of the pelvis. Softened by the effects of
relaxin, this joint relaxes and opens up a little to
allow the birth of your baby. Many pregnant women
also experience pain in the back of the pelvis, often
deep in the buttocks. This unpleasant sensation
may occur only in one side or may seem to move
from one side to the other.

You may also experience pain when walking,
climbing stairs, standing from sitting, turning over
in bed, getting out of the car, separating your legs,
or standing on one leg—perhaps while dressing or
getting into a bath. The pain is often worse at night,
especially after an active day.

What you can do about it Follow all the recommendations on pages 130–131, but also:

- Ask your physician if physical therapy (page 178) or another form of therapy (see *What Might Work?*, page 176) would help, and ask for a referral to a qualified practitioner. Make sure that the practitioner you choose is experienced and qualified in matters to do with women's health, and, in particular, problems in pregnancy.
- Avoid slumping in your chair, sofa, or bath.
- Avoid any heavy lifting—and don't push any heavy shopping carts or baby strollers.
- Rest—the amount of pain you feel can be directly related to how active you've been, so rest for at least 10 minutes every hour.
- Sit down to dress, iron, and do other chores.
- When turning over in bed or getting up from standing, pretend your knees are glued together and move both legs as a single unit.

After your baby's born Back pain can continue after your baby has been born, particularly as you lift and feed him or her. But you can reduce the chances of postnatal back pain if you take sensible precautions. Follow the general advice on lifting and carrying on pages 152–155, and take note of the following special tips:

- Go to postnatal classes to strengthen your stomach and pelvic floor muscles—and generally get back into shape.
- Pay attention to your posture (page 148).
- Make sure your back is supported, especially when feeding your baby.
- Lift your baby (or older child) correctly with your back straight, hugging your baby close to the center of your body. Your feet should be apart,

with one leg slightly in front of the other. Then lift using your leg muscles. To put your baby down, reverse the procedure. To practice the movement, do the "goblet squat" (page 167).
- When putting your baby in a car seat, try not to bend over. Instead, place the baby on a seat close to the door, maintaining your hold, then climb in so that you do not have to bend and twist at the same time. Try bending your knees and resting them on the door rim.
- Carry your baby on your front or back whenever possible. If carrying on one side, alternate sides.

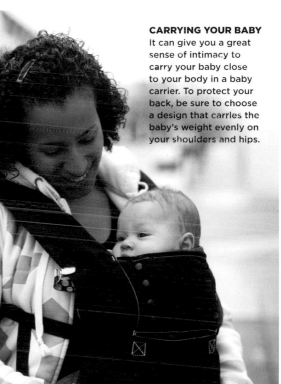

CARRYING YOUR BABY
It can give you a great sense of intimacy to carry your baby close to your body in a baby carrier. To protect your back, be sure to choose a design that carries the baby's weight evenly on your shoulders and hips.

Use these exercises to combat minor aches and pains that are caused by minor muscle strains or ligament sprains. Do each exercise in turn and finish by repeating the pelvic tilt. Be sure to check out the cautions on page 10.

Pelvic tilt

1 Lie on your back in the neutral position (page 25) with your knees roughly at right angles. Place your hands behind your head to support your neck, or place a pillow under your head.

2 Arch the small of your back—your lumbar spine—away from the mat, but keep your buttocks on it.

3 Then lower the small of your back, pushing it down toward the mat. Repeat 10 times in a slow, controlled rhythm. Finish in the neutral position.

Seated tilt

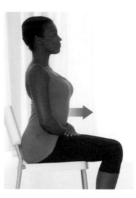

1 Sit upright on a hard chair in the neutral position (see Step 3). Increase the forward arch of the small of your back to move it away from the chair back.

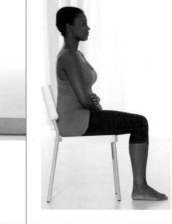

2 Then slouch down, rounding your lower spine. Repeat Steps 1 and 2 ten times in a slow, controlled rhythm.

3 Finish with a forward arch (as in Step 1) and return to the neutral position (pictured).

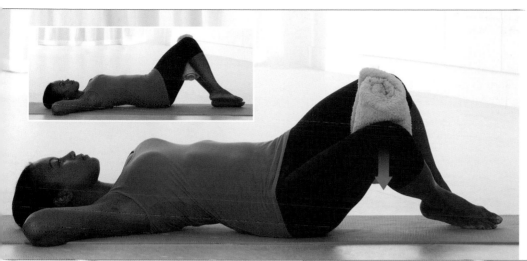

Towel roll

Lie on your back with your knees bent at right angles and place a rolled-up hand towel between your knees. Rock your knees from side to side as far as is comfortable. Repeat 10 times.

Buttock lift

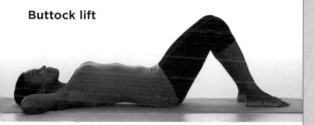

1 Lie on your back with your knees bent at right angles and your feet shoulder width apart.

2 Lift your buttocks off the mat. Hold for 30 seconds, then lower. Repeat five times.

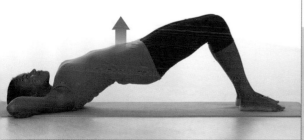

Curl-uncurl

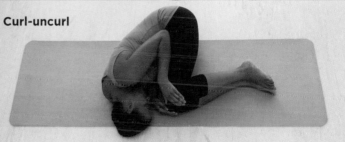

1 Lie on your side on a mat and curl up into a ball, making yourself as small as possible. Hold for 30 seconds.

2 Then uncurl, arching your back, with your hands above and behind your head and your legs back. Repeat the sequence five times.

These exercises are useful for easing aches and pains in the middle part of your back, such as pain between the shoulder blades and any pain that may be felt when breathing deeply. Before doing these exercises, be sure to check with your physician if you have a current back problem, and read the cautions on page 10.

Diaphragmatic breathing

1 Lie on your back with your knees bent at right angles and a pillow under your head to support your neck, then relax. Rest your hands at the bottom of your rib cage, with your fingers just touching below your sternum (breastbone).

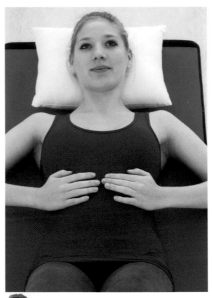

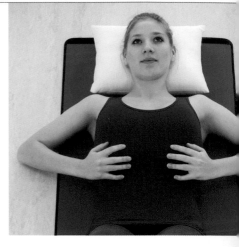

2 Inhale deeply through your nose, filling your lungs—you should feel your fingers separate and your ribs expand. Hold the breath for a few seconds, relax, and exhale. Repeat three times. Rest, and repeat twice more.

Seated twist

1 Sit on a hard chair with an upright back.

2 Reach your left hand down the front right leg of the chair as far as possible. Hold for 10 seconds and then straighten slowly. Repeat five times.

3 Repeat Step 2 on the other side.

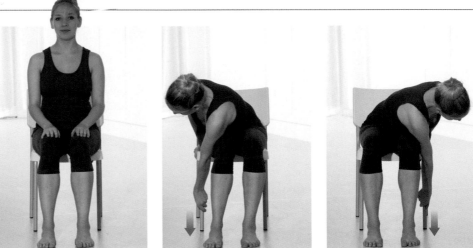

Shoulder-blade squeeze

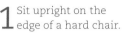

1 Sit upright on the edge of a hard chair.

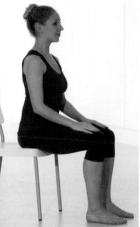

2 Bend your elbows at right angles, then pull your elbows behind you, squeezing your shoulder blades together. Hold for 10 seconds.

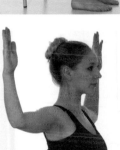

3 Bring your arms forward and wrap them around you—as if hugging yourself—pulling your shoulder blades apart. Hold for 10 seconds and relax. Repeat five times.

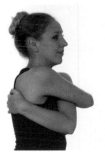

Lateral twist

1 Lie on the floor with your knees bent and your head supported by a pillow. Place both arms straight up behind your head. Relax and hold for 30 seconds.

2 Raise your arms so they are in a vertical line with your shoulders.

3 Stretch your right hand over toward the left as far as possible without lifting your right hip off the ground. Hold for 10 seconds and then lower your arms. Repeat on the other side. Do the full sequence five times.

Both sciatica and pirformis syndrome have similar symptoms, which often involve severe pain. The exercises on these pages can help relieve the pain of both conditions; those on page 139 specifically stretch the piriformis muscle. Read the cautions on page 10 before you start.

Sciatica relief position

Lie on the floor with your hips and knees at right angles and your lower legs resting on a stool or chair.

McKenzie acute sciatica exercise

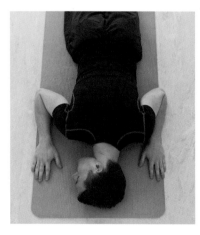 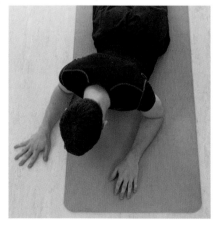 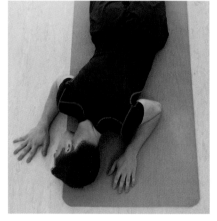

1 Lie on your stomach on the floor or a hard bed with your arms bent and hands close to your shoulders.

2 Lift up so that you are resting on your elbows. Relax. Check whether the pain moves toward your buttocks. If not, move to one side, then check again, and if not, move to the other side.

3 If you find a position that moves the pain as described, relax and hold the position for three minutes. Repeat frequently—up to every two hours—but never hold any position that is painful.

Diagonal knee grasp

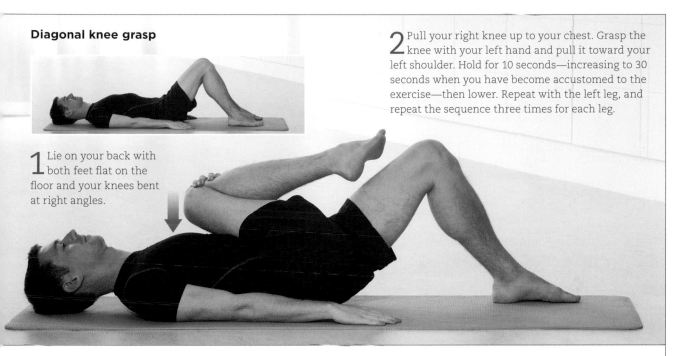

1 Lie on your back with both feet flat on the floor and your knees bent at right angles.

2 Pull your right knee up to your chest. Grasp the knee with your left hand and pull it toward your left shoulder. Hold for 10 seconds—increasing to 30 seconds when you have become accustomed to the exercise—then lower. Repeat with the left leg, and repeat the sequence three times for each leg.

Ankle-on-knee stretch

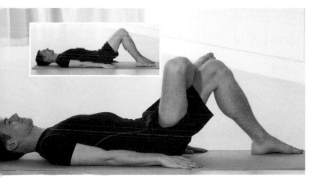

1 Lie on your back with both feet flat on the floor and your knees bent at right angles. Place the ankle of your right leg on your left thigh.

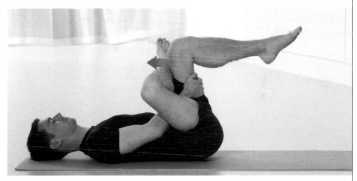

2 Pull your left leg up to your chest and hold for 10 seconds—increasing to 30 seconds over time—and then lower. Repeat with the left leg and repeat the full sequence three times.

Sacroiliac Joint Exercises ▸▸

These exercises help to relieve sacroiliac pain. But remember that you should consult your physician first to find out the reason for your problem. Otherwise the trouble will recur. Also check out the cautions on page 10. Use a thin cushion to support your head and neck if you need it for comfort.

Fist squeeze

1 Lie on your back with your knees bent at right angles.

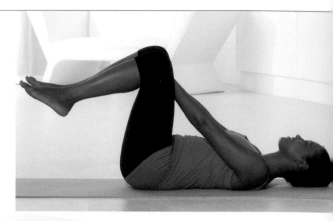

2 Place your fists between your knees. Keeping your back flat on the mat, raise your feet. Squeeze your knees together and hold for 10 seconds. Repeat five times.

Reverse squeeze
From the starting position shown in Step 1 (above), place your hands on the outside of the knees. Push your knees outward against the pressure of the hands and hold for 10 seconds. Rest, then repeat five times.

Scissor push

From the starting position shown in Step 1 (opposite), raise your feet off the floor. Place your right hand on the top of your right knee and your left hand under the left knee. Hold for 10 seconds, then push your right knee against the resistance of the right hand at the same time as you push your left knee against the left hand. Repeat five times and then reverse hand positions and repeat the sequence.

Knee over body

From the starting position shown in Step 1 (opposite), bring the right leg over to the left side. Use your left hand to increase the stretch. Hold for 10 seconds. Repeat five times, then repeat the exercise with your left leg.

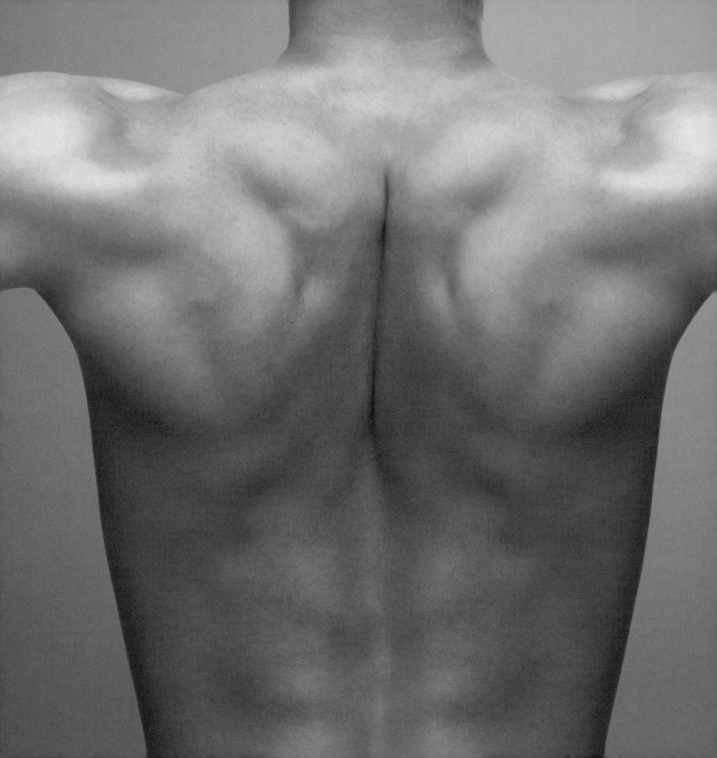

Chapter 5

The Healthy Back

This amazing structure, with its complex engineering, needs careful maintenance from an early age to give you the best chance of lifelong back health. This chapter contains vital advice on how to achieve good posture and how to protect your back while undertaking everyday activities. There are also tips on maintaining a healthy weight and on dealing with stress in the interests of back health. And there's a series of healthy back exercises to help you stay pain free.

Stable, Supple, and Strong

A healthy back is one that combines stability, flexibility, and strength. And to get that kind of a back you need strong vertebral bones, strong deep muscles and ligaments, and efficient intervertebral disks. Fortunately, if you exercise regularly but gently, you can get precisely that.

Strong abdominal muscles add to the security and stability of the spine. Apart from their other functions, they maintain the correct intra-abdominal pressure, which helps relieve pressure on the intervertebral disks, and reduces the likelihood of forward slippage of one vertebra over its neighbor. When you bend over, contracting them, the intra-abdominal pressure rises even further so that the abdominal contents are raised within the cavity, taking pressure off the base of your spine. In addition, the muscles are vital in maintaining good posture (page 148).

Also important are the numerous small "core" muscles that attach to each bony protuberance of the vertebrae, running horizontally, vertically, and diagonally. They contract and relax to maintain the correct curvature of the spine (page 149) and allow each spinal segment to move a little on its neighbor.

Keep it moving Flexibility is vital for good spinal health, because it allows you to perform everyday activities easily, and reduces the risk of injury or pain. In order to lead a normal life, you need to be able to bend, stretch, and twist. If you don't have—or regularly use—the full range of available movement, joints stiffen and their muscles weaken.

Flexibility is joint specific, which means that you can have an excellent range of movement in one joint, but be severely limited in another. The problem is that one tight, inflexible joint can put undue pressure on its neighbor—for example, tight hip flexors at the hip joint can increase the lumbar curve (page 52) and lead to low-back pain.

In all cases, the watchword for prevention is "keep it moving." Anyone, of any age, can improve and maintain flexibility by practicing correct stretching techniques (page 164). You should stretch all your joints fully—and especially those of your spine, shoulders, and hips—at least three times a week. But be careful, especially when embarking on a new exercise program. Never push through pain, and don't "bounce" with jerky, up-and-down movements as doing so can tear muscle, tendon, and ligament fibers, causing muscles to go into spasm to protect both themselves and your joints, which leads to rigidity. The best way to maximize the exercise benefit and avoid strain is to stretch to a point of mild discomfort, ease back slightly, then hold that position for a minute.

Strong muscles in the back and abdomen provide stability, protect the spine from injury, and reduce the stress placed on spinal bones and joints. But these muscles require regular exercise to maintain strength and tone. While muscles such as the gluteals—the muscles in your buttocks—are used every time you walk or go upstairs, your back and abdominal ones are often underused and weak because of our sedentary lifestyles.

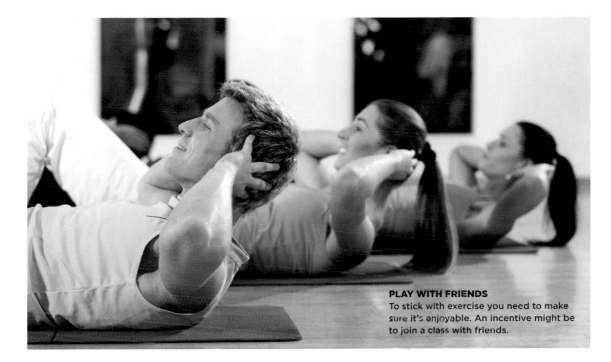

PLAY WITH FRIENDS
To stick with exercise you need to make sure it's enjoyable. An incentive might be to join a class with friends.

How to get what you want Work your back and abdominal muscles by doing the strength exercises, starting on page 169 at least three times a week, working them a little harder each time. Give them a day off between workouts to avoid injuries.

Another problem is that we all spend too much time sitting and slouching over—whether at workstations, while driving a car, or watching TV. This puts considerable downward pressure on the vertebrae and squashes the intervertebral disks (page 16), leading to a greater risk of injury, especially in the lumbar spine. Spending prolonged periods sitting down leads to shortening of key muscles and ligaments and this can lead to permanent stiffness. And, of course, age plays its part in reducing flexibility.

THE GOOD, THE BAD . . . AND THE UGLY

Exercise is necessary for health, but some activities are better at promoting a healthy back than others. Here are some examples of activities that can be roughly classified as the good, the bad, and the ugly. Just keep in mind that whichever activity you choose, it's vital that you follow the rules of good posture (page 148) because incorrect posture will undo any benefits of "good" exercise activities and worsen the ill-effects of "ugly" ones. And check out the specific exercises to give you a healthy back, starting on page 164.

The good The following simple activities help prevent back problems from developing by keeping your spine flexible and increasing muscle strength.

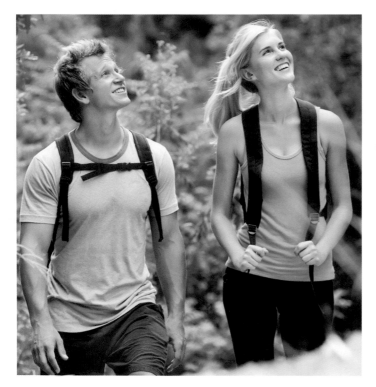

Swimming is particularly good if you're pregnant. But remember: the crawl and backstroke are the best strokes to use because they lengthen the muscles and increase flexibility; don't do a flip turn at the end of each length; don't extend your neck too far back when you breathe; swim gently and rhythmically to avoid straining your neck and lower back.

- **Yoga** A gentle yoga class (page 196) can promote a healthy back by increasing flexibility, strength, endurance, balance, and posture. The key word here is "gentle": hatha yoga is the most suitable type. More vigorous disciplines, such as ashtanga or power yoga, can cause back problems or make them worse. Take things at your own pace, don't overstretch, and make sure that you choose a good teacher.
- **Pilates Method** An increasingly popular exercise technique (page 192), Pilates exercises strengthen the deep postural muscles that support correct alignment of the spine and helps correct any muscle imbalances, thereby decreasing wear and tear on the spinal joints. Pilates also improves the strength and flexibility of the muscles and teaches awareness of any bad movement habits.
- **Dance** This excellent form of exercise improves posture, maintains strong bones, increases muscle strength and stamina, and increases balance and co-ordination. It's fun, too. Which dance style is right for you depends on your age, fitness, whether there is any existing back problem— and your inclination. Start slowly and build up gradually until your fitness levels have improved.

The (possibly) bad It may be a bit unfair to call all these activities "bad," because their potential to damage your back depends largely on how you do them. But caution is certainly warranted.

WALKING BACK TO HEALTH
Walking is an ideal form of exercise for back health. It promotes circulation and boosts the strength and flexibility of the spinal muscles. Just be careful to carry any gear you need in a well-designed backpack that spreads the load evenly over your shoulders.

- **Walking** This activity eases muscle tension, encourages continuous interaction between the muscles, stretches the connective tissues, promotes healthy blood circulation, and deepens breathing. Concentrate on walking with good posture, relaxed shoulders and neck muscles, and a loose-limbed gait.
- **Swimming** A low-impact activity that takes pressure off your spinal joints and muscles, it gives you a good cardiovascular workout, tones your stomach and back muscles, and increases flexibility.

- **Jogging** An excellent way to stay fit and maintain bone strength, but the high impact of running, especially on hard surfaces, can place stress on the spinal joints of the lower back. To minimize your chances of an injury, remember that it is vital to warm up first (page 96). Start and end by walking, then jog slowly, building up speed. When you've finished, give your spine a good stretch out to open up your impacted lower spine. If you experience back pain, you should probably consider another aerobic activity.
- **Golf** Walking around a golf course can be a wonderful way of exercising, as long as you don't have a heavy bag of clubs to carry—if you do, swap shoulders between each hole or, better still, use a cart. Even so, a golf swing and a stooping posture are not good for your back. Counter them by stretching your back after every stroke and doing practice swings the other way around.
- **Cycling** This is a good general exercise to improve fitness that strengthens your hip and leg muscles. But stooping over the handlebars on a racing bike is not good. The forward-flexed position shortens your hip flexors and puts a lot of strain on your lower back and neck. If you cycle in this position, take time to stretch your hip flexors and back muscles and strengthen your gluteal and stomach muscles. "Sit-up-and-beg" bikes are far better for your back—and static bikes that have back supports are better still.

The ugly These activities carry a risk to your back if not undertaken with care.

- **Tennis, racquetball, and badminton** All these racket sports have pluses and minuses. A plus is that the outcome is increased fitness and stamina and the maintenance of bone strength. Minuses

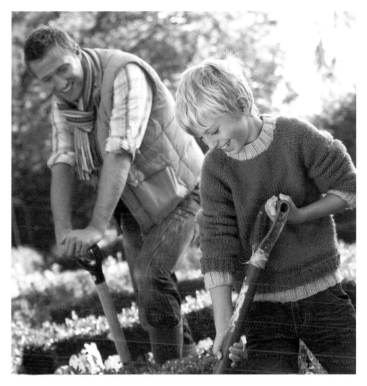

include the fact that they involve twisting and bending, often under strain. They also develop one side of the body more than the other, so putting unnatural stresses and strains on the spinal column. To avoid this, exercise the "opposite" side to achieve a balance.

DIGGING DEEP
Gardening can be a great way of getting exercise in the fresh air while doing something useful. But be sure to alternate spadework with rest and tasks that are less "back-stressful" such as pruning or dead-heading.

- **Gardening** Gardening can put considerable stress on your back. The secret of minimizing these stresses is to think "little and often." Alternate heavy work that involves stooping, such as digging and weeding, with light chores. And take frequent breaks to rest and stretch your spine.

Take the Right Posture

Adopting a standing, sitting, or walking posture that places minimum stress on your spine and other supporting structures is one of the key contributions you can make to the health of your back. On these pages we'll show you what good posture is and how to improve and maintain it in your daily life.

The Southern California Orthopedic Institute defines what the word "posture" means extremely well: it is "the body's alignment and positioning with respect to the ever-present force of gravity. Whether we are standing, sitting, or lying down, gravity exerts a force on our joints, ligaments, and muscles. Good posture entails distributing the force through our body so no one structure is overstressed."

We are all familiar with the image of a soldier standing to attention: eyes front, shoulders back, stomach and backside in. But does it demonstrate good posture? The answer is "no." The soldier may look great, and the various parts of his or her body are certainly in their correct positions. But the body is rigid and taut, which breaks one of the prime rules of good posture: your body must always be loose and flexible, held in what physical therapists call a "neutral" position.

Good posture means holding your body in such a way that pressures over joints are even and natural, and muscles are not stretched or tensed. Anything else causes muscle tension, and puts strain on the joints. So your spine should be straight, when looked at from the back. But when looked at from the side it should be showing its natural curves. Any deviation from this suggests increased and perhaps uneven pressure on individual areas, stretched ligaments, and tense or stretched muscles.

Why posture matters The reason why pressure over joints should be even and natural and muscles should be relaxed, not tense or stretched, has to do with the fact that there are two types of muscle: phasic and postural. Phasic muscles contain a high proportion of fast-twitch fibers—that is, the muscle fibers that act and react the most quickly—and are the muscles you use to make a deliberate action. Postural muscles, with a high proportion of slow-twitch fibers, are at work all the time, keeping the body upright and in its correct position.

If your posture is poor, and the various parts of your body are not positioned correctly relative to each other, one group of postural muscles will be taut and the opposing muscles will be over-stretched. As a result, neither group works efficiently, and with time the stretched muscles become weaker, leading to postural misalignment and an increased risk of back problems. For example, if your lumbar spine is too arched, your abdominal muscles will be over-stretched and their opposing muscles will shorten and become tense.

Be posture aware A key part of any strategy for preventing or recovering from back problems is to know what good posture looks and feels like. The information and illustrations on the following pages will help you do that.

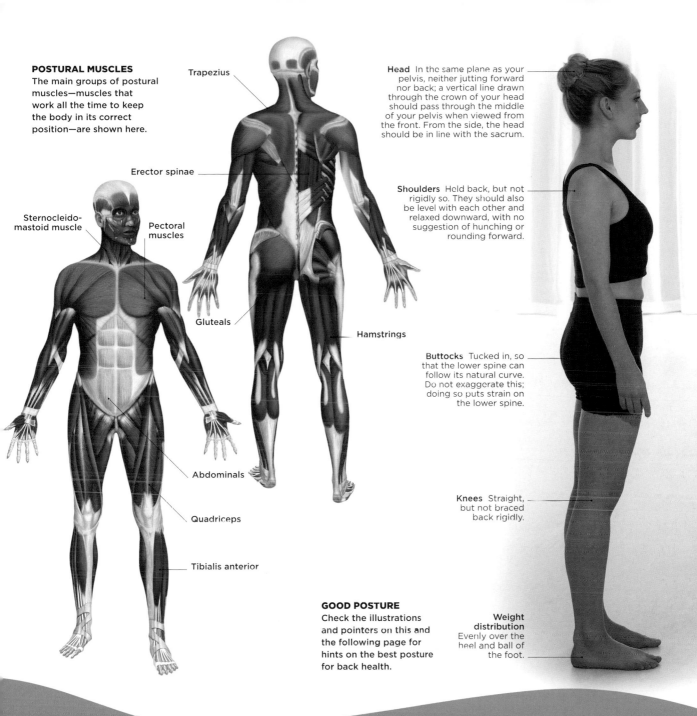

POSTURAL MUSCLES
The main groups of postural muscles—muscles that work all the time to keep the body in its correct position—are shown here.

Trapezius

Erector spinae

Sternocleido-mastoid muscle

Pectoral muscles

Gluteals

Hamstrings

Abdominals

Quadriceps

Tibialis anterior

Head In the same plane as your pelvis, neither jutting forward nor back; a vertical line drawn through the crown of your head should pass through the middle of your pelvis when viewed from the front. From the side, the head should be in line with the sacrum.

Shoulders Held back, but not rigidly so. They should also be level with each other and relaxed downward, with no suggestion of hunching or rounding forward.

Buttocks Tucked in, so that the lower spine can follow its natural curve. Do not exaggerate this; doing so puts strain on the lower spine.

Knees Straight, but not braced back rigidly.

Weight distribution Evenly over the heel and ball of the foot.

GOOD POSTURE
Check the illustrations and pointers on this and the following page for hints on the best posture for back health.

Make the crown of your head its highest point Push it toward the ceiling, so that you elongate your neck, but avoid any tension.

Look straight ahead Neither up nor down.

POSTURE ADJUSTMENT
Stand in your underwear in front of a long mirror. If you have long hair, pile it on top of your head so that you can see your shoulders, neck, and earlobes.

Hold your chin in a straight, neutral position Not sticking up or tucked in.

Keep your neck straight Neither tilted to one side nor the other.

Hold your shoulders back and down Not hunched or rigid.

Maintain your natural spinal curves (page 14), both in the upper and lower back Make sure that no more than the usual muscle tone is needed to keep the vertebrae in place and undue pressure is not put on joints and ligaments.

Balance your body Any variation of the spine from the vertical can cause great strain on joints and muscles. So make sure your body is balanced vertically: your shoulders and hips should be level, with your arms hanging loosely by your sides and your head balancing comfortably on your neck.

Is your posture damaging your back? The first step to good posture is honest observation. Stand in front of a mirror and look at yourself critically. Assess your posture according to the key posture pointers highlighted at left.

First of all, try to put your head in the correct position (as described left). Then ask yourself the following questions:

- **Is your head tilted one way or another or are your shoulders crooked?** If they are, your trapezius muscle (page 76) may be too tight on one side and too stretched on the other. This may be a sign of scoliosis (page 54), a sideways curvature of the upper spine, but is often the result of overuse of the muscles on one side.

- **Are your shoulders hunched up and tense?** If so, your neck muscles will almost certainly be tense as well, causing strain on the neck region of the spine (cervical spine) and shoulder joints, and giving rise to tension headaches.

- **Are your shoulders rounded and does your chest curve in?** If so, you will probably notice that the palms of your hands face too far back. Your chest muscles are likely to be too tight and your upper back muscles will be overstretched. Women may find that their breasts have a tendency to sag. This imbalance can impair breathing efficiency and perhaps reduces the amount of oxygen you are able to inhale and the amount of carbon dioxide you exhale.

- **Are the tips of your hip bones crooked and pointing too far forward or backward?** Unfortunately, you may have a scoliosis (page 54) of the spine. If the tips of your hip bones are too far forward, you probably have hyperlordosis (page 56)—an accentuated curve of your lumbar spine—that causes your back muscles to tighten, your abdominal muscles to become less effective, and your bottom to stick out. If the tips of your hip bones are too far back, you may suffer from the opposite problem, and have an overly flat back, an equally damaging fault. This often leads to the head being ahead of the pelvis when viewed from the side and, in some cases, a protruding stomach. Both problems can affect the way in which weight is transferred by the lumbar spine, putting strain on the joints between the vertebrae.

- **Are your kneecaps pointing outward or inward?** Your knees should be level and the kneecaps pointing forward. If they point outward you may well suffer from bowlegs; if inward, you may have knock knees. Both problems can affect the way in which weight is transferred down the leg and cause problems in the lower back, hips, knees, and in the arches of the feet.

- **Do your feet point outward or inward?** People whose feet point outward from the midline often suffer from a fallen medial arch—"flat feet." But low-back, knee, hip, and foot problems are likely to be the result whether your feet point either inward or outward, because weight is no longer distributed efficiently through the foot when walking or standing.

Hold your head up! The position of the head and neck provides the key to good posture. If your head is in the correct position, your shoulders tend to fall into place naturally and there is a feeling of balance and harmony.

If your head is not in the correct position, the muscles of the neck and upper back have to stretch and tense constantly in an attempt to adapt to the unnatural position, and the result can be neck pain and headaches.

How Good Posture Helps ▸▸

By maintaining good posture you can:

- Reduce the chances of suffering from headaches, neck pain, backaches, and arm pain.

- Make movements more precise and less stressful on muscles and joints.

- Reduce both physical and emotional tension and stress.

- Permit more efficient breathing, that may increase your oxygen intake and boost your energy levels.

- Give a positive, confident impression to others.

You probably move your head more than any other part of your body, as you look at things and talk to people, so it is vital to get into the habit of holding your head correctly even while you are moving it.

Getting into the habit Good postural habits do not come easily, especially if you spend much of your time seated, staring at a fixed point—looking at a computer screen, for example, or while driving for long periods. When you're busy or tired, it's all too easy to let your head sag forward and your neck twist, and your back to sag. The only way to change your habits is to focus on them and continue to do so until your body has learned new habits and correct posture becomes automatic.

On the following pages you'll find plenty of tips for adopting a healthy posture in your everyday life—at work and in the home.

How to Avoid Strain

If you make an effort, it's not too difficult to keep posture in mind when you're walking from place to place or moving from task to task. The difficulty comes when you're stuck in one position for some time or when you are carrying out a task that has unusual physical demands.

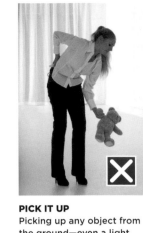

PICK IT UP
Picking up any object from the ground—even a light one—can strain your back if you don't do it correctly. Always bend your knees and keep your back straight.

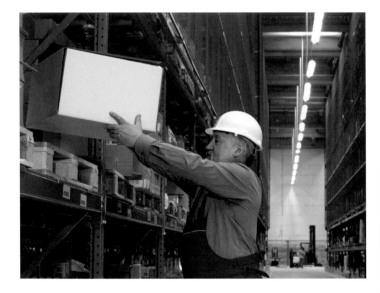

Keep your back straight

Bend your knees

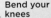

BACK STRAIN AT WORK
Many types of work involve the possibility of back strain, but jobs involving lifting and carrying are among the highest risk occupations for back injury.

From heavy manual work to desk work, waiting tables, and everyday tasks in the home, most activities have areas of potential risk for your back. But most hazards in your work or home life can be controlled if you keep in mind these three basic rules: choose the correct equipment; use the correct technique; and take regular breaks. The following pages have general tips that you can use in many situations.

Bending down When loading a washing machine, putting a dish in the oven, or just picking up a toy from the floor, make sure that you bend your knees rather than your back.

LIFTING SAFELY

Incorrect ways of lifting can be bad for your back, because you're using the back muscles to do work for which they're not designed. So when lifting:

- Keep your back straight and use the muscles of your legs.
- Place one hand underneath the object, if possible, and pull it close to your body. It's worth remembering that a weight held at arm's length increases the stress on your spine by up to *10 times* that of the weight itself.

Heavy objects It's a great temptation to just stoop down and grasp a heavy object in order to lift it. But if you do this you're putting yourself at considerable risk of damaging your back.

Instead, stand with one foot slightly in front of the other as close as possible to the object to be lifted. If you can, keep both feet flat on the floor. Bend your knees and hips until you are low enough, keeping your back straight. Straighten up in one smooth movement, using your hip and leg muscles and keeping your back straight. Only start to move once you're standing erect.

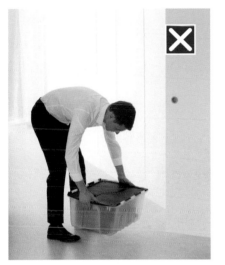

RIGHTS AND WRONGS OF LIFTING
The photograph above shows a lifting position that carries a high risk of back strain: the person has reached down with a bent back and straight legs. A much safer position is shown right: he has lowered himself by bending the knees and has kept his back straight. Far right, he carries the heavy object close to his body to reduce the amount of strain.

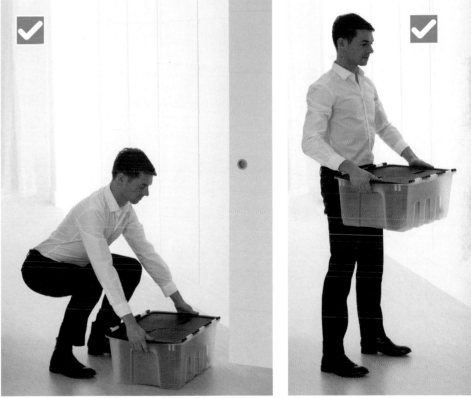

IN THE HOME

Research suggests that women whose only exercise is housework are often as fit as those who work out at a gym. This is probably because, like gym exercises, much housework involves bending, stretching, pushing, and pulling. Unfortunately, housework can also place considerable strain on your back and encourage poor posture. Here are a few pointers on how you can reduce the risk of postural problems and injuring your back.

Vacuuming Hold the handle of your vacuum cleaner high enough so that you do not have to bend over. Hold it close to your body, so that you use your feet to move it around rather than bending and stretching.

Work surfaces Whether at a kitchen counter or at the ironing board, the height of the work surface should allow you to stand with a straight back while you're working.

Keep your back straight

Bend your knees

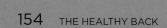

VACUUMING SAFELY
Always avoid movements that involve bending while pushing. Whatever type of vacuum cleaner you use, keep a straight back and lower yourself when necessary by bending your knees.

WORK AT THE RIGHT HEIGHT
The key to avoiding back strain while ironing is to have your ironing board at a height that allows you to stand up straight.

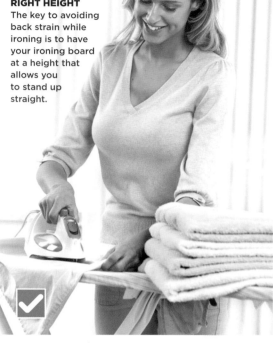

IN THE YARD

Yardwork can expose your back to a variety of risks, most of them the result of unusual stresses on the postural muscles. To avoid such problems:

- Always use the tools that are right for you—check their weight and balance before you buy.
- Use a long-handled hoe or weed wacker to dispose of weeds.
- Always go down on your knees to plant.
- Never swing a hover mower in arcs—and always work directly behind the mower.
- Do not dig for longer than 30 minutes without a break—and warm up with some low-back exercises (page 134).

BACK-FRIENDLY GARDENING
Your mantra should be "straight back and bent knees" for all ground level tasks such as planting and pulling up weeds.

DESK SENSE
Whenever you sit at your desk, consciously check your posture. If you follow the posture tips on this page, you will avoid the back-straining posture errors shown right, and instead will soon get into the habit of the healthy deskwork position pictured below.

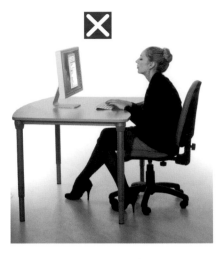

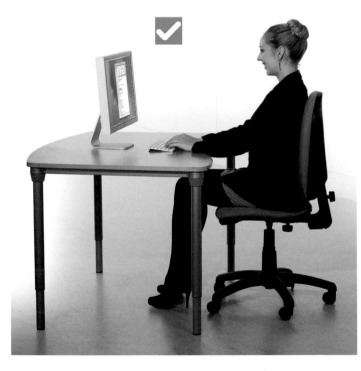

AT YOUR DESK

Many of us have jobs that involve sitting at a desk for long periods, often using a computer. This necessarily imposes a fair amount of strain on the back, neck, and shoulder muscles. So it is vital that your chair helps to support these areas. Its backrest should be adjustable, so that it can be maneuvered to support the lumbar region of your spine, and any chair that has a full-length backrest should have an additional support area at this level.

Chair adjustment Your chair should be deep enough from front to back to support most of the length of your thighs, and its seat should be tilted forward and downward to an angle of five degrees from the horizontal. This should allow your thighs to rest at 90 degrees when your feet are flat on the floor. Your screen should be positioned so that it faces you directly and you do not have to look downward at it, which puts strain on the extensor muscles of the neck. And when you are reading for long periods, use a reading stand if at all possible.

Your position Let your hands fall naturally onto the keyboard with your elbows and forearms supported, on armrests if necessary. This means that your chair has to be higher than if you were writing at a desk. You will probably need one that has a height-adjustment mechanism to make this possible—such chairs are more expensive than normal ones, but are worth the investment.

Take a break It is important that you take frequent breaks from your computer, too, because as well as easing any tension in your postural muscles, taking a break will reduce the risk of strain injury, upper limb disorders, and eyestrain. Short, frequent breaks are generally best. Try to take a five-minute break

Keep High Heels for Special Occasions ▸▸

Shoes did not play a part in our evolution—in fact, they are a relatively recent development, evolutionarily speaking. In their early days, shoes were worn for comfort and protection, but now for many of us they are now as much a fashion accessory. Which is where high heels come in.

The unfortunate truth High heels are very bad for your back: they wreck your posture by pushing your center of gravity forward and so increasing the curve of your lumbar spine. This puts pressure on your spinal joints, ligaments, and supporting muscles, and may also have an effect on the spinal nerves, which can lead to pain in the lower back and down the back of your leg known as sciatica (page 118).

High heels are bad for your feet and calves, too: a spokeswoman for The American Podiatric Medical Association says that wearing high heels is "shoe-icide." So keep them for special occasions. On most days wear a heel no higher than two inches (5 cm).

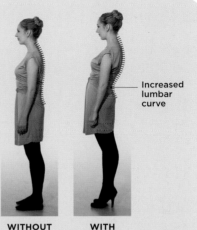

Increased lumbar curve

WITHOUT HEELS   **WITH HEELS**

every half hour or so. Walk around while loosening your shoulders and rolling your neck to release any tension and stretch your back.

IN THE CAR

Whether you are a driver or a passenger, long car journeys can wreak havoc on your back. This is especially true if you tilt your seat back. Your lumbar spine then has to bear too much of your body weight. It's vital that you sit correctly, and it's easiest to do so if your seat is kept upright.

Choose a car with seats that help maintain this upright position and have a lumbar support. The base should not slope down at the back or too much weight will be borne by the base of your spine, rather than by your thighs. The backrest should support your whole trunk.

Even with the correct car seat, immobility can build up tension in your back muscles. Avoid this problem by taking frequent breaks. Get out of your car every hour and move around, then do some stretches to relieve tension in your neck and shoulder muscles. If you feel that you are tensing up in your car, breathe evenly and deeply, allowing tension to drain away, and try to consciously relax your shoulder muscles with each exhalation.

A SUPPORTIVE SEAT
To prevent strain during long journeys, a car seat should be firm, adjustable, and supportive. Lumbar supports are excellent.

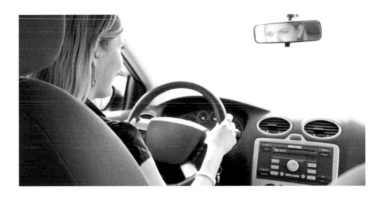

Lighten Up

It's just common sense: carrying too much weight puts greater strain on the joints in your back and makes them more prone to damage. Not only do the additional stresses increase general wear and tear but they also make the back more vulnerable to other problems, such as strained ligaments and compressed disks.

How being overweight affects your back

Overweight people, and particularly men, tend to carry much of their extra weight in the abdominal area, which increases the stress on the spine more than extra weight in the legs and buttocks. Overweight people also often have weak abdominal muscles, which provide inadequate support for the spine. Without good muscular control, the spine is much more vulnerable during any strenuous activity such as lifting or carrying. Normally, when they're tense, the abdominals increase the pressure within the abdominal cavity so the cavity itself can take some of the weight-bearing role, which relieves stress on the spine. Here's how excess weight can cause problems for your back:

- Extra pounds cause poor posture—an increased lordosis (page 52)—so that your weight is not borne centrally by your disks and vertebrae.
- Extra pounds cause the early onset of osteoarthritis (page 58), due to excessive wear and tear.
- Extra pounds cause flattened disks that are prone to prolapse—"slipped disk" (page 15)—and which also lose their ability to act as shock absorbers.
- Extra pounds flatten the intervertebral disks, causing a reduction in the space between the vertebrae, putting pressure on the facet joints (page 16). Any movement increases the friction in these joints, which become inflamed and painful.
- Extra pounds increase wear on the spine, which together with weak abdominal muscles, makes the back an inadequate scaffold for lifting. And that increases the likelihood of back problems.

If you suffer from a back problem and are overweight, it's vital that you reduce your weight through sensible eating and exercise.

It's just plain common sense.

GET ACTIVE Boosting the amount of exercise you take is a vital component of any weight-loss program. But get medical advice first.

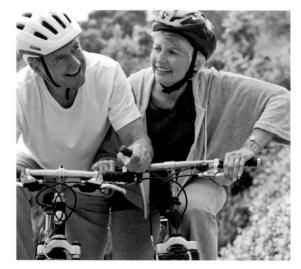

Am I Overweight? »

The standard reference that doctors use to judge whether a person's weight is healthy is BMI (body mass index). This is a calculation based on your height and weight, which provides a useful guide for most people. But BMI can be inaccurate for those who are well muscled but lean, as well as for those who have little muscle bulk in proportion to body fat. Check this table for a quick guide to whether your weight is healthy or if you need to take action.

Underweight

Healthy

Overweight

Obese

Very obese

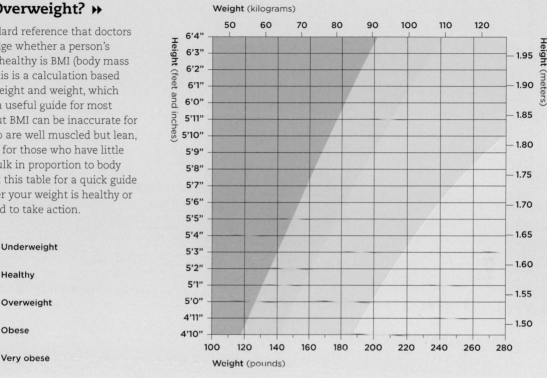

How to lose weight sensibly Faddy diets often work in the short term but not in the long term. So here are some tips for losing weight and not regaining it:

- Aim to lose no more than 2 pounds (1 kg) a week.
- Check your calorie intake. The recommended daily intake ranges from 1,600 calories for a sedentary woman over 50 to around 3,000 calories for a man in his 20s or 30s in a physically strenuous job. To lose weight but give your body the fuel it needs to function, you should never let

your calorie intake fall below 1,000 (women) or 1,500 (men) calories a day. Further information is available in *Dietary Guidelines for Americans,* on the U.S. Department of Health and Human Services website (http://health.gov).
- Don't try crash dieting: the body responds to starvation by slowing down the rate at which you burn calories. Such diets can lead to severe malnourishment and muscle wasting.
- It's better to eat little and often—up to four or five times a day—than to have just one or two large meals a day.

- If you find yourself craving food between meals, restore your blood sugar levels by eating complex (unrefined) carbohydrates, such as a slice of wholegrain bread, rather than a candy bar.
- Serve your food on smaller plates—portions won't look any smaller than they did before—and avoid snacking by eating only at the table.

HOW MANY CALORIES DO I NEED?
Daily calorie needs depend on your gender, age, and importantly, your activity level. Use this table, based on the recommendations of the 2010 Dietary Guidelines Advisory Committee, to check your calorie needs.

- Maintain your awareness of weight and diet by weighing yourself daily and writing down what you eat every day.
- Beware of slimming pills and "miracle" weight loss programs. Check with your doctor before taking any type of slimming aid, particularly if you are taking other medication.

Take care Dieting unwisely can be as harmful as unhealthy eating, so:

- Plan to lose weight gradually, not overnight, to avoid depriving the body of essential nutrients.
- Adopt a less restrictive diet after you have reached your ideal weight. If you find this hard, consult your doctor.
- If you have serious difficulty in keeping your weight down, consult your doctor. You may have a problem that requires medical treatment.

Advised Daily Calorie Intake ▸▸

Age (years)	Male			Female		
	Sedentary	Moderately Active	Active	Sedentary	Moderately Active	Active
18	2,400	2,800	3,200	1,800	2,000	2,400
19-20	2,600	2,800	3,000	2,000	2,200	2,400
21-25	2,400	2,800	3,000	2,000	2,200	2,400
26-30	2,400	2,600	3,000	1,800	2,000	2,400
31-35	2,400	2,600	3,000	1,800	2,000	2,200
36-40	2,400	2,600	2,800	1,800	2,000	2,200
41-45	2,200	2,600	2,800	1,800	2,000	2,200
46-50	2,200	2,400	2,800	1,800	2,000	2,200
51-55	2,200	2,400	2,800	1,600	1,800	2,200
56-60	2,200	2,400	2,600	1,600	1,800	2,200
61-65	2,000	2,400	2,600	1,600	1,800	2,000
66-70	2,000	2,200	2,600	1,600	1,800	2,000
71-75	2,000	2,200	2,600	1,600	1,800	2,000
76+	2,000	2,200	2,400	1,600	1,800	2,000

Feed Your Back ▸▸

There's no need for a special diet for back health
Your back will get the nutrients it needs from a normal healthy diet—that is, one that contains plenty of fresh fruit and vegetables, whole grains, low-fat dairy produce, and fish and lean meat (or an alternative vegetarian source of protein). The healthy eating plate below shows the proportion of foods from these different groups that you should aim for.

Are vitamin supplements necessary? For most people, taking multivitamin and mineral supplements is unnecessary. Even so, many of us don't get enough calcium and vitamin D for optimum bone health, not just for dietary reasons, but because we are not sufficiently exposed to sunlight, which is vital to vitamin D production. Look at the section on osteoporosis (page 68) to see what supplements are recommended.

What about glucosamine and chondroitin? Taken separately or as a combined pill, there is some evidence that these supplements reduce joint pain in osteoarthritis (page 58), but since they affect mainly cartilage, of which there isn't much in the spine, the evidence is limited when it comes to backs. Most doctors will tell you that buying these supplements is a waste of money.

And omega-3? Several small-scale studies have shown that omega-3 fatty acid (fish oil) supplements are as good as NSAIDs (page 204) at relieving back pain, and they're certainly a lot safer. So far, the jury is out—but since they have other benefits, too, they may be worth a try.

Always ask your doctor Before making any major changes in your diet or taking any vitamin, mineral, or other nutritional supplements.

Fruit and vegetables (excluding potatoes)

Bread, rice, potatoes, pasta, and other high-carbohydrate foods

Meat, fish, eggs, beans, and other non-dairy sources of protein

Milk and dairy products

Foods and drinks high in fat and/or sugar

Be Relaxed

Muscular tension is the enemy of good back health. It places extra stresses on the spine, stretches the ligaments, and distorts body posture—which, in turn, leads to back problems. But you can ease this muscular tension by practicing some simple relaxation techniques. And they will soothe your mind and spirit!

The fight or flight response Stress and relaxation are opposite sides of the same coin, and both are necessary for a healthy life. For early humans, how quickly they reacted to a threat could be, literally, a matter of life or death. The stress response (opposite) developed to cope with any threat quickly and efficiently, so that the body was

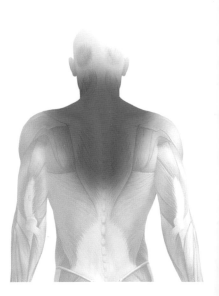

MUSCLE TENSION
Typically, stress causes tension in the neck and shoulder muscles.

Five-Minute Back Relaxation ▸▸

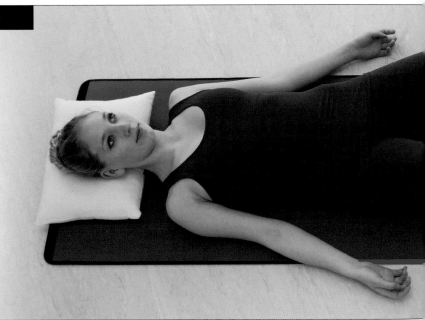

This position takes the pressure off your lumbar spine and sacroiliac joints. Supporting your knees on a foam roller (pictured) or resting your legs on a chair reduces strain.

Take deep breaths while you concentrate on relaxing areas of tension starting with your feet and working up through your legs, buttocks, and arms. In each area, first tense the muscles, hold for a few seconds, and then relax. Then hunch and drop your shoulders. Finally, gently rock your neck from side to side. Rest for 15 minutes.

prepared to take rapid action—whether to fight a saber-toothed tiger, say, or, more sensibly, to flee from it. One way or another, the situation was soon resolved, the stress response then died down and the body returned to its previous, relaxed state.

Most modern threats cannot be resolved by a physical response. You cannot run out of a meeting that you feel is going badly, for example, or punch the boss—if, that is, you wish to keep your job. You cannot run from a traffic jam or a supermarket line, unless you are willing to lose your car or your groceries. And the lack of a clear resolution means that it is all too easy to be in a constant state of stress, with our muscles remaining tense and ready to act at a moment's notice but never acting. The solution? To shut down the body's stress response by using relaxation techniques.

A network of tension The back, neck, and shoulders are the areas of the body most likely to be affected by muscle tension because of the intricate network of deep muscles that support the spine (page 18) and provide core stability. Unfortunately, when that network gets tensed, the result can be headaches, aches and pains, general tiredness, and poor posture (page 148).

Focus within The technique described (left) reduces the accumulated stress in the back, by progressively contracting and relaxing the muscle groups that store tension. But to succeed, one important lesson should be kept in mind: the essence of relaxation is to bring focus inside ourselves, so that we become aware of the tensions within specific muscles. This allows us to consciously relax each and every one, which helps to relieve the pain and tiredness caused by muscular tension.

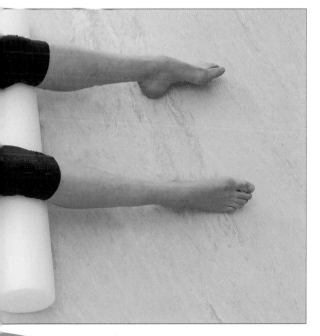

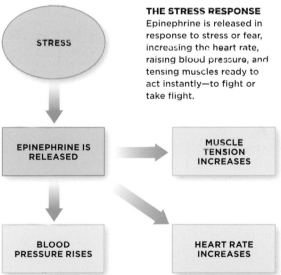

THE STRESS RESPONSE
Epinephrine is released in response to stress or fear, increasing the heart rate, raising blood pressure, and tensing muscles ready to act instantly—to fight or take flight.

STRESS

EPINEPHRINE IS RELEASED

MUSCLE TENSION INCREASES

BLOOD PRESSURE RISES

HEART RATE INCREASES

Sitting down for long periods shortens the muscles that flex the hips (the iliopsoas and the quadriceps) and the hamstrings, which places a significant amount of extra stress on the lower back. These stretches lengthen the muscles, giving greater flexibility. As a result, your back is better safeguarded from injury—when, for example, you bend to pick up an object from a low table. Before doing these exercises, be sure to check with your physician if you have a current back problem, and read the cautions on page 10.

Seated hamstring stretch

1 Sit on a mat with both legs straight out and feet flexed.

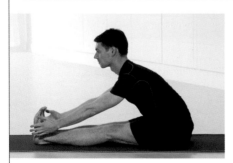

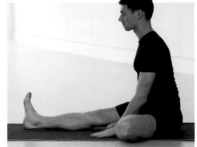

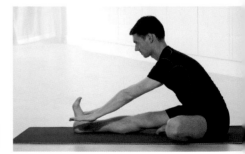

2 With a straight back, bend forward at your waist and stretch your arms as far as you can toward your feet, without going through any pain. Keep your knees straight. Hold for 30 seconds, then relax. Repeat five times.

3 Sit on the floor with one leg straight out and the other bent so that the sole of that foot is resting against the inner thigh of the straight leg.

4 Bend at the hips and stretch your arms out over the straight leg toward your foot. Hold for 30 seconds, then repeat five times.

Wall push

1 Stand facing a wall with your arms straight out in front at shoulder height. Place your hands shoulder-width apart on the wall.

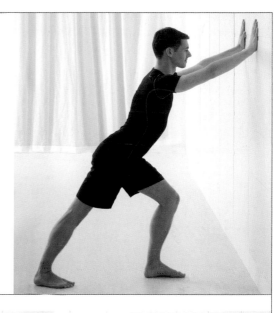

2 Take a step back with one leg while pushing your body into the wall. Keep your back straight and both heels down. Hold for 30 seconds, then repeat five times. Repeat the sequence using your other leg.

Hip hinge

1 Stand with your feet shoulder-width apart and your knees slightly bent.

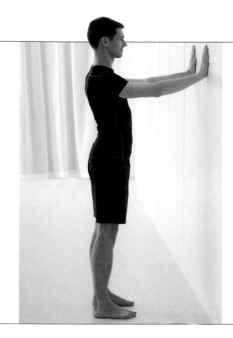

2 Keeping your back straight and your knees still, push your buttocks out and bend forward at the hips—do not round your back— until your torso is at right angles to your legs.

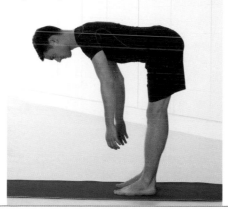

3 Stand up straight by tightening your buttock muscles and pushing your hips forward in one smooth movement. Repeat five times.

Quad stretches

1 Stand next to a support—a chair back or a tabletop, say—for balance.

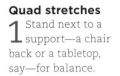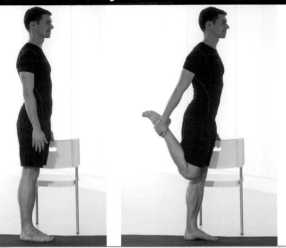

2 Bend one knee up behind you and grasp your foot with your hand, then pull the knee as far back as possible. Hold for 30 seconds and repeat five times. Repeat the sequence with the other leg.

3 Lie on your stomach on the floor resting on your forearms.

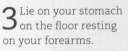

4 Bend one knee back as far as it will go without pain and bring the hand on the same side back to hold your foot. Hold for 30 seconds, then repeat five times. Repeat the sequence using your other leg.

Movement Exercises for a Healthy Back ▸▸

These exercises increase both lower back and abdominal core strength, and promote your positional awareness so that you are less likely to damage your back. Each exercise should be performed slowly and with attention to detail. And before and during each exercise you should check that your spinal curves are natural and correct. Before doing these exercises, be sure to check with your physician if you have a current back problem, and take note of the cautions on page 10.

Goblet squat

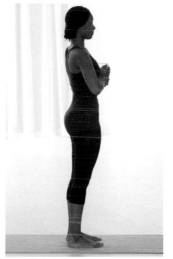
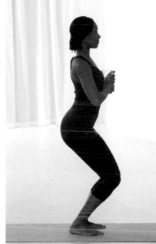

1 Stand up straight with your feet shoulder-width apart and slightly turned out. Hold a glass half-full of water with both hands against your chest.

2 Then bend your knees, sinking down as far as you can by pushing your buttocks back. Keep your head facing forward, your back straight, and your chest up to avoid spilling any water. Hold for 10 seconds and then rise back up. Repeat five times.

Hands to knees

1 Lie on your back with your knees up and bent at right angles, and with your hands by your side and your neck still.

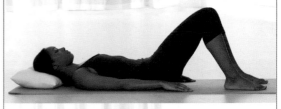

2 Stretch forward with both hands to touch your knees. Hold for 10 seconds, then lower slowly. Repeat five times.

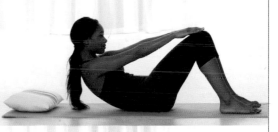

3 Next, reach forward with your right hand to touch the outside of your left knee. Hold for 10 seconds and lower. Then repeat, moving your left hand to your right knee. Repeat both movements alternately five times each

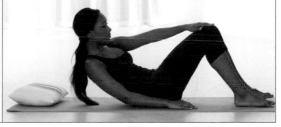

Exercise ball work

1 Lying on your back on a mat, place an exercise ball on your stomach and grasp it with both hands and knees.

2 Release the ball with one hand and the knee on the opposite side—to do this, let the hand drop behind your head and lower the opposite knee. Hold for 10 seconds, then grasp the ball again and repeat with the hand and knee on the other side. Repeat the sequence five times.

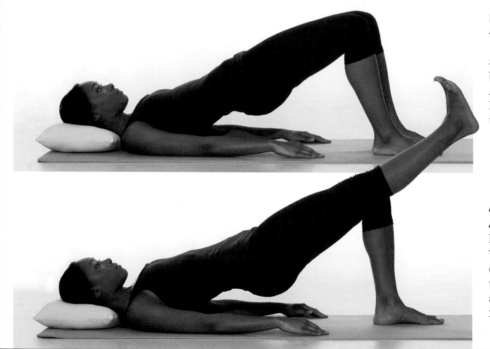

Buttock lift

1 Lying on your back with your knees bent at right angles, raise your buttocks off the mat. Aim to achieve a straight line from your shoulders to your knees.

2 Lift and straighten each leg alternately, holding for 10 seconds. Then lower your buttocks down to the mat. Be sure that your lower back is in a neutral position (page 25). Repeat five times.

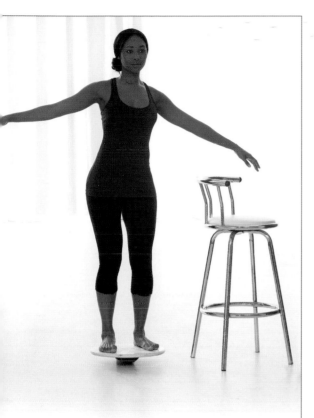

Wobble fit

Use a wobble board (if you do not have one, try standing on a plump cushion to start with and progress to using two plump cushions). Place the wobble board close to a chair back or table that you can grasp for balance if necessary. Stand on the board with your feet shoulder-width apart and try to maintain your balance for as long as you can—you should aim to build up to five minutes over time. As the exercise becomes easier, put your feet closer together; and later try standing on one leg and then the other.

The exercises below and on the next page help increase the strength of the muscles that support your back. Increased strength helps increase your mobility and protects you from injury. Before doing these exercises, be sure to check with your physician if you have a current back problem, and observe the cautions on page 10. The side pull (below) uses a resistance band. This is a popular exercise aid that often come in packs of three, each one having a different level of resistance. Start at the lowest level of resistance and work up.

Side pull

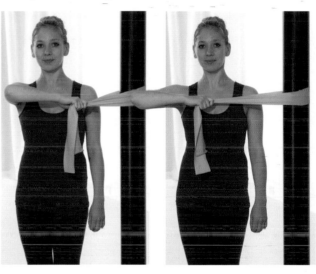

1 Place a resistance band around a post or banister at shoulder height and, standing sideways to the post, grasp both ends with the far hand so that the band is taut but not stretched.

2 Pull the band in to the center of your chest. Hold for 10 seconds, making sure that you do not allow your body to twist, then release slowly. Repeat five times, then turn to face the other side and repeat the sequence.

The plank

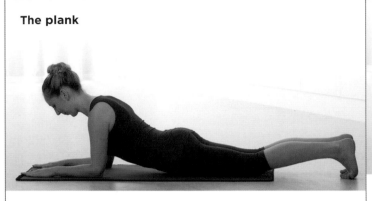

1 Lie face down on a mat with your elbows under your shoulders.

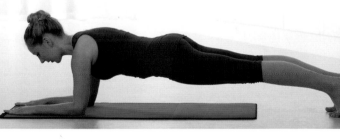

2 Push your whole body up off the floor in one smooth motion, so that you are supported by your toes and lower arms. Make sure that you keep your trunk straight. Hold for up to 10 seconds, then lower slowly. Repeat five times. It may be necessary to build up to a 10 seconds hold and it is better to do one plank correctly—with a straight spine—than more incorrectly.

Walking the dog

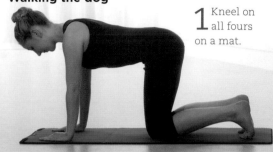

1 Kneel on all fours on a mat.

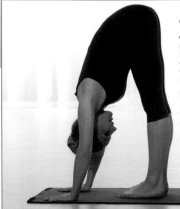

2 Straighten your knees and lift your buttocks. Allow your head to drop between your arms.

3 Walk your feet toward your hands. Then walk your hands away from your feet to return to the Step 2 position. Repeat this sequence five times.

Stretch and curl

1 Kneel on all fours facing the floor, with your knees and hands, directly under your hips and shoulders respectively.

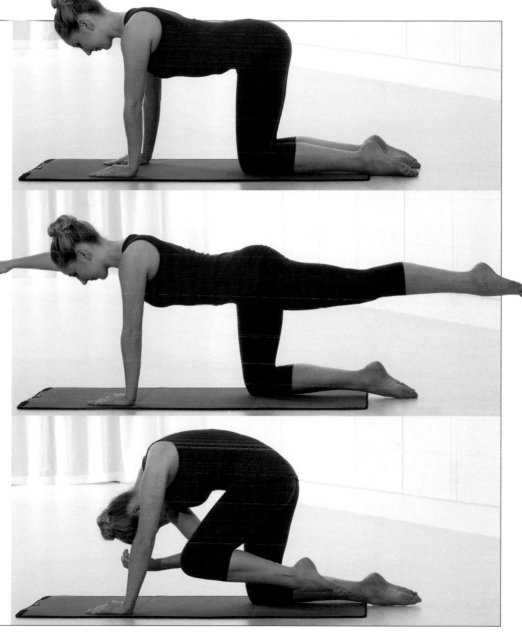

2 Lift your right hand and left leg off the floor and stretch out. Hold for 10 seconds and then lower slowly.

3 Round your back and bring your right hand and left leg under your body. Repeat on the other side. Repeat the sequence five times. If you feel that the movement is not fully under control, start by lifting one hand, then one leg and so on, until you can balance properly.

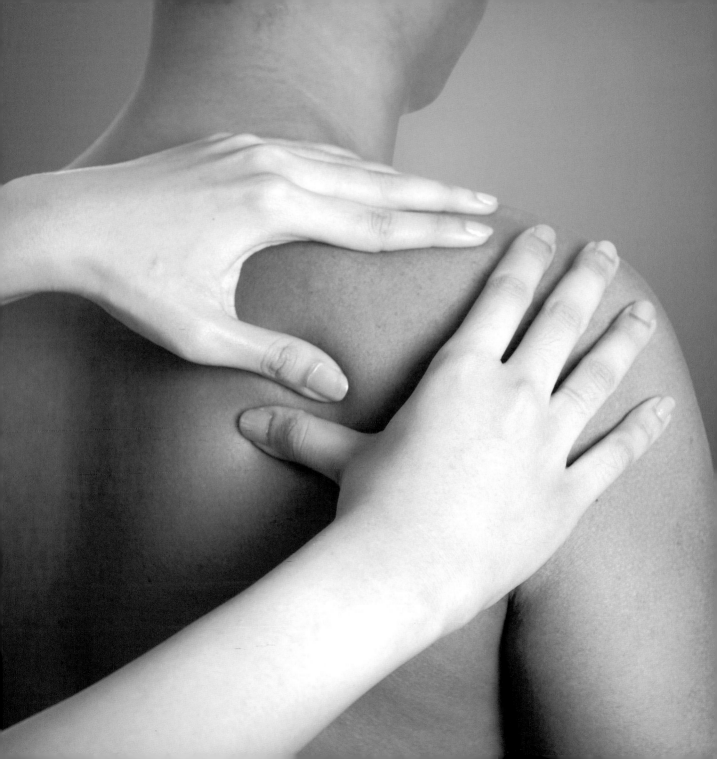

Chapter 6

Glossary of Treatments

Here you'll find clear descriptions of the mainstream treatments your physician may recommend as well as information about the most widely used complementary therapies. From physical therapy to chiropractic and massage, and from medication to acupuncture and spinal surgery, the principles and risks of each form of treatment are explained.

The Right Treatment—for You

Every back problem, just like those who experience them, is unique. That's why, in the vast majority of cases, there is no single "right" treatment that will be the best choice for everyone. In this chapter you'll find out about a variety of treatments to help you decide, along with your healthcare provider, what's right for you. Here are a few tips on making your choice.

Be an expert patient Apart from in the exceptional case of a serious accident, when decisions are likely to be made by those providing emergency care, you will be involved in making choices about your treatment plan. Numerous studies have shown that those who participate in decisions around their healthcare can expect a more positive outcome.

Much depends on the nature and severity of symptoms, your age and general health, and not least on your personal preferences. But the message is: whatever kind of back problem you have, learn about it so that you can work in partnership with your physician to determine the right treatment approach for you. And if you don't feel up to making this effort, ask a family member or close friend to help.

Ask questions When you visit your physician to discuss treatment options, it's all too easy to forget to ask the questions that you need to have answered. So it's a good idea to write down any questions and take a notepad and pen to the doctor's office. That way you can note key pieces of information, which often get forgotten. And if you think it would help, take a friend or relative with you—both to provide moral support and be an extra pair of ears. Some of the questions you might like to ask include:

- What's the precise name of my condition?
- What are the treatment options?
- How good are their chances of success?
- What are the possible side effects or risks?
- How long before I can expect to feel better?
- What can I do to help myself?

Think In many cases your physician will have a clear idea of what would be the best treatment plan for you. To feel confident with this decision, you'll need to think through the pros and cons of the treatment options. In particular, you should consider the possibility of side effects. And, with surgery, you'll need to balance the potential benefits with the risks. A second opinion is always a good choice.

Ask for a referral In most cases, your physician will put you in touch with any specialists that you need to see—for example, a spinal surgeon. But if you think additional advice could be helpful, don't be afraid to ask for a referral to another professional. In particular, if you think complementary therapies could work for you, ask your physician if he or she can recommend a qualified practitioner.

IT'S A JOINT DECISION
You and your medical advisers are partners in the quest for the right treatment for you. Be sure to ask the questions—and get the answers—you need.

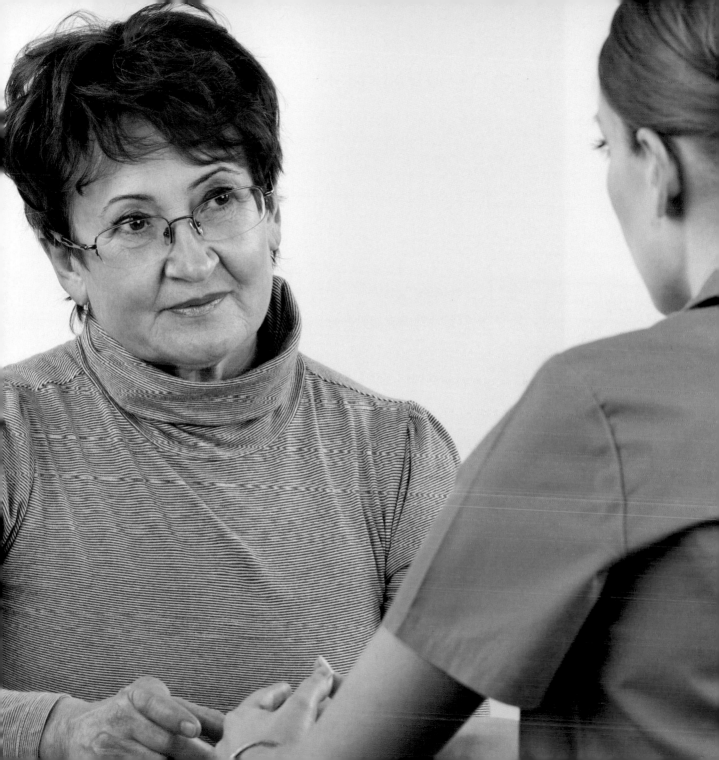

What Might Work?

In this chapter you'll find descriptions of the main treatment options, and this table will give you a broad idea of what might be appropriate in your case. But your treatment will depend on many variables, so follow your physician's advice, which is based on in-depth knowledge of you and your health needs.

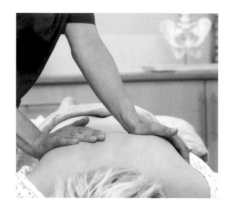

KEY
●●● Common primary treatment or therapy
●● Possible back-up treatment or therapy
● Treatment or therapy that may provide benefit or may relieve symptoms

TYPE OF PROBLEM ▼	TREATMENT/THERAPY ▶ Physical therapy	Osteopathic medicine	Chiropractic	Massage therapy
Posture problems	●●●			●●
Spinal curvatures	●●	●●	●●	●●
Osteoarthritis	●●●			●●
Rheumatoid arthritis	●●			●●
Anklyosing spondylitis	●●●			
Osteoporosis	●●●			
Soft-tissue Injuries of the neck and upper back	●●●	●●●	●●	●●●
Nerve root problems of the neck or back	●●●	●●	●●	
Thoracic outlet syndrome	●●●	●●	●●	
Shoulder muscle injuries and inflammation	●●●	●●	●●	●●
Ligament sprains and tears	●●●	●●	●●	●●●
Rehabilitation from injuries (including fractures)	●●●	●●	●●	
Soft-tissue injuries of the middle and lower back	●●●	●●●	●●●	●●●
Disk degeneration	●●●	●●	●●	
Spinal stenosis	●●●			
Sciatica	●●●	●●	●●	
Sacroiliac joint problems	●●●	●●●	●●●	●
Piriformis syndrome	●●●	●●●	●●	●
Pregnancy	●●●	●●●		●

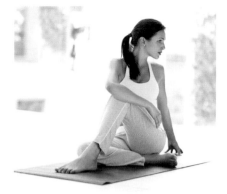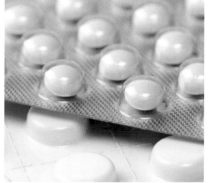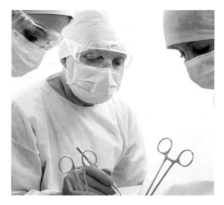

Alexander Technique	Pilates Method	Yoga	Acupuncture	Shiatsu	TENS	Medication	Surgery
●●●	●●●	●●●					
●●	●	●					●●●
		●●	●●			●●●	●●
		●			●	●●●	●●
●	●●	●●				●●●	●●
	●●	●●				●●●	
●●	●	●	●	●	●	●●●	
			●	●	●	●●●	●
●●					●	●●●	
	●	●	●	●	●	●●●	
						●●●	●
					●	●●●	●●●
●●●	●●	●●	●●	●	●●	●●●	
					●	●●●	●●
						●●●	●●●
			●	●	●	●●●	●●
●●	●●	●●	●		●●	●●●	
●	●	●	●	●	●	●●	
●●	●●	●●	●	●		●	

Physical Therapy

Physical therapy is often the cornerstone of treatment for a range of back problems that cause pain and limit movement. It is delivered by a physical therapist (PT) and deals with any physical dysfunction or injury that prevents the body from functioning to its full potential, using a personalized program of therapeutic exercises and other techniques.

What you can expect Physical therapists work in many settings, such as hospitals, clinics, schools, workplaces, and sports centers. Depending on where you live (see below), you can either see one by self-referral or following a referral from a physician.

A PT will look at your medical history and the results of any medical tests, together with any physician's report, before conducting a thorough physical examination. This may involve asking you to perform a variety of physical movements. After making an assessment, your PT will devise an individual treatment plan, following recommendations that are called "protocols." With orthopedic PTs—the ones who treat back problems and provide back rehabilitation programs—this usually includes exercises, postural education (page 148), and general lifestyle advice, such as on lifting (page 152), and relaxation techniques (page 162).

The initial assessment and treatment normally lasts at least an hour; subsequent sessions are likely to last between 45 minutes and an hour. Wear loose, comfortable clothing so that you can move easily. Most therapists' offices try to ensure that you are seen by the same PT at each visit.

How it works An important part of any PT treatment is a full explanation of what the problem is, what can be done about it, what the treatment program entails, and how it can help. Your program is likely to consist of some or all of the following:

Exercise There are three main types of exercises used in PT treatments: active, passive, and isometric. Active exercises—ones that you perform yourself—are the most frequently used, especially if you have a back problem. You will be prescribed graded exercises that are initially performed under your PT's supervision, and extended into a home exercise routine.

Where Do You Live? ▸▸

In 46 of America's states, you can refer yourself to a physical therapist for treatment. But in Alabama, Indiana, Michigan, or Oklahoma it is against the law to see a PT for treatment without a doctor's prescription. In Michigan and Oklahoma, though, you are free to see a PT without a prescription, but only to have an evaluation—the PT will send a report to your doctor, who will decide whether treatment is appropriate (and so can be justified to your health insurer).

Unfortunately, life can also be complicated in the other 46 states as well, depending on your health insurer. Some will pay for treatment without a doctor's prescription; others will not. So check before you make an appointment.

In passive exercises the PT, rather than you, moves your joints through their full range of movement to ease joint swelling, relieve tension, and promote mobility. Isometric exercises—in which the joint in question remains still—are used when movement produces pain or muscle spasm, or to maintain muscle strength. You will be asked to contract the appropriate muscle without causing any movement, hold the contraction and then relax the muscle.

"The McKenzie method" is also used. Robin McKenzie, a physical therapist in New Zealand in the 1960s, realized that when your spine is lengthened, any pain from the upper limb or leg often "centralizes" to the neck or lower back. Mackenzie method exercises aim to lengthen the spine and relieve the focus of the pain (a McKenzie exercise is shown on page 138). An advantage of this method is that, after the PT has prescribed an exercise routine, you can manage your own back problem and return to your normal routine. The method is not suitable where pain does not "centralize" or if you have spinal stenosis (page 116) or osteoarthritis (page 58).

Mobilizations and manipulations Mobilizations are gentle repetitive pressure movements performed by the PT to restore full range of movement, loosen joints, and ease muscle spasm. Manipulations are more forceful movements to correct the alignment of the spine. There are two types of spinal manipulation and mobilization:

■ **Maitland's mobilizations** Geoffrey Maitland, an Australian PT, developed a system of passive mobilizations (during which the patient does nothing) that is used throughout the world. Mobilizations are a manual therapy designed to restore your range of movement by gently

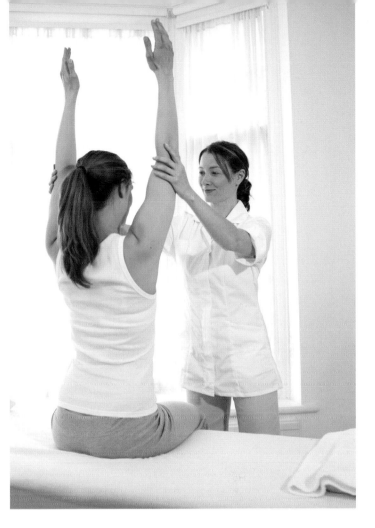

easing a joint so as to achieve its full mobility. The technique is used on both synovial and nonsynovial joints (see page 17). Maitland stressed that every patient needs a careful and thorough evaluation before treatment, and that the treatment itself should be tailored by the information gained from continual assessment by the physical therapist.

INITIAL ASSESSMENT
Your physical therapist will check your range of movement and physical alignment to help determine an appropriate program.

■ **Mulligan's mobilizations**
Brian Mulligan, a New Zealand PT, built on Maitland's mobilizations and developed the concept of spinal mobilizations that are "sustained natural apophyseal glides" (SNAGS), focused on the facet joints (see page 16). SNAGs involve a gliding mobilization of an affected joint by the PT with a simultaneous corresponding movement by the patient. After a few repetitions, you will be asked to make the movement on your own to discover if your range of pain-free movement has increased.

Cold Cold packs are usually the first thing a PT uses. The application of cold can reduce local inflammation, swelling, bruising, and pain.

Heat Heat can relieve pain, muscle spasm, and stiffness, and increase blood flow to an area of the back. A PT can apply heat to the affected tissues by various means: heat lamps, heat compresses, hot lotions, and sprays warm the superficial tissues to ease muscle tension and spasm; short-wave and microwave diathermy machines aim to heat the deep tissues by means of electromagnetic waves, although the scientific basis for this is unproved.

Ultrasound An ultrasound machine emits high-frequency sound waves that are inaudible to the human ear. The waves penetrate the skin—they're completely painless—and help fight the local inflammation that is caused by many back problems, relax muscles that are over-tight or in spasm, and so relieve pain.

Aquatic therapy Aquatic therapy consists of an exercise program that is performed in warm water under the supervision of a physical therapist. Water provides buoyancy and support for the body, minimizing weight-bearing pressure on the joints, and is especially useful for people who suffer from problems affecting the lower back because the supportive effect of water permits the patient to perform exercises that might be too painful to try on dry land.

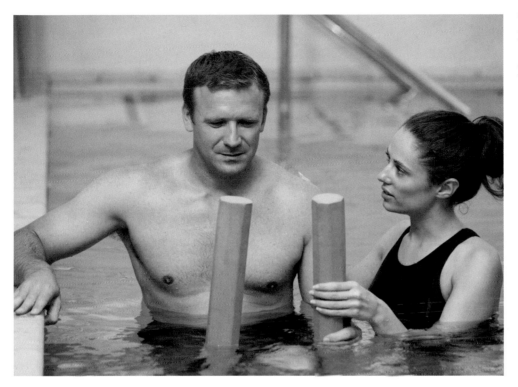

TAKING THE PLUNGE
A PT will often get into
the pool with the patient
in order to be able to give
effective guidance and help
with necessary adjustments.

One of the benefits of exercising in water is that it provides a certain amount of resistance, so that muscles can be strengthened without the need for weights. The end result for most people is an improvement in muscular strength, endurance, balance, coordination, and positional awareness. And the warmth of the pool—normally kept at 84–92°F (29–33°C)—eases pain and dilates blood vessels, which helps increase the circulation and encourages the muscles to relax, thereby increasing the flexibility of the spinal joints. Salt water is often used for aquatic therapy, because it increases buoyancy and is thought by some practitioners to have an additional painkilling effect.

Put in Practice ▸▸

To be able to practice, physical therapists must have a qualification accredited by the Commission on Accreditation of Physical Therapy Education (CAPTE) and be licensed by the state in which they practice. They must also undertake continuing education to maintain their license. By 2016, all PTs must have doctorate degrees, and will be styled DPTs.

PTs often specialize in specific body systems, so there are respiratory, pediatric, cardiac, and neurological physical therapists. But many become orthopedic PTs, specializing in the musculoskeletal system. So check that the PT you choose has the necessary experience to treat your condition.

Osteopathic Medicine

In common with the practitioners of many complementary therapies, osteopathic physicians believe that each part of the body is interconected. While fully trained in all aspects of medicine, they often use osteopathic manipulations in their treatment.

Doctors of osteopathic medicine (DOs) also believe that the human body is self-regulating and has the ability to heal itself—that it strives to adapt and maintain itself in a state of balance termed homeostasis. They believe that stress, injury, poor diet, or other factors can upset the balance, and illness and disease are the result.

It's all connected If the musculoskeletal system is not kept correctly aligned, DOs believe that the performance of all other body systems will be affected. Another important concept in osteopathic medicine is that of "dysfunction." If you hurt your lower back, for example, you may stand awkwardly and stiffly. But even after the injury has healed, you may still stand that way, especially when you're over-tired or stressed. So a DO will assess your posture, how you move, and the way you breathe to check for any dysfunctions.

Acceptance Gained »

Osteopathy is a treatment approach that was devised by Andrew Taylor Still, an American engineer and medical doctor, in the late 19th century. In 1972, osteopathic physicians, who had attended osteopathic medical schools and known as DOs, were recognized in the U.S. as medical doctors.

Today, all DOs in the U.S. have full medical qualifications as well as osteopathic ones. Their certifying body is the American Osteopathic Association.

Fixing the problem An osteopathic physician may prescribe a whole range of conventional treatments, including medication and surgery. But depending on what is challenging your health, he or she is also likely to give lifestyle advice and use hands-on techniques known as osteopathic manipulative treatment (OMT) that may include:

- **Soft-tissue manipulation** Also called myofascial treatment, this is a form of massage that usually involves stretching of muscles, tendons, ligaments and joints, and the application of deep pressure. It can be superficial or deep, and either fast or slow. It eases stiffness and tension, relaxes the muscles, and stimulates circulation.
- **Articulatory techniques** Designed to increase the range of movement, articulatory techniques involve the DO moving joints through their full range of movement to stretch shortened muscles, ligaments, and other stiffened soft tissues. The movements are often rhythmical.
- **Traction** In this technique two joint surfaces are pulled slightly apart. It is used to loosen joint capsules, ligaments, and the surrounding muscles and tendons. A small, springing movement may be used on certain joints that have little inherent movement, such as the spinal joints or sacroiliac joint, in order to increase the range of movement and stretch the ligaments.

The Evidence ▸▸

A number of studies have demonstrated that osteopathic manipulative treatments are a valuable way of treating low-back pain. Many non-osteopathic medical doctors agree that such treatments are useful, especially for preventing acute back pain from becoming chronic (page 36), but many remain unconvinced that OMT can have any effect on body systems other than the one causing a problem.

- **High-velocity/low amplitude techniques (HVLAs)** These fast, abrupt, thrust manipulations are perhaps the best known OMT. A joint is pushed gently to the limit of its range of movement followed by a fast, downward thrust. This moves it outside its normal range for a short time and can cause the gas bubbles in the synovial fluid (page 16) to burst with an audible "crack." These manipulations may be uncomfortable for a moment or two, but they are rarely painful.
- **Muscle-energy techniques** These are used for both diagnosis and treatment. The patient moves a part of the body against resistance provided by the DO. When a barrier to continued, smooth motion is sensed by the DO, the patient stops the movement. At this point, the patient is asked to pull away from the barrier and return to the movement's starting point while the DO resists the movement. This encourages the muscles involved to relax and lengthen. These techniques are particularly useful when more vigorous thrust techniques may not be advisable, as, for example, in those who are frail or elderly.

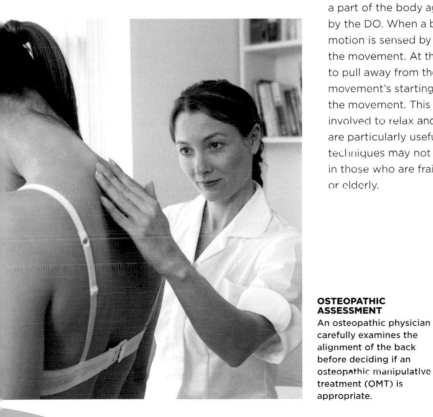

OSTEOPATHIC ASSESSMENT
An osteopathic physician carefully examines the alignment of the back before deciding if an osteopathic manipulative treatment (OMT) is appropriate.

How to Keep Your Balance ▸▸

Maintaining osteopathic homeostasis—a state of balance is something you can learn to do yourself. Just keep these four basic principles in mind:
- Maintain good posture.
- Exercise.
- Learn how to relax completely.
- Eat a healthy diet.

Chiropractic

Founded by Daniel David Palmer in 1895, chiropractic is a therapy that has survived many years of bitter struggle with the orthodox medical establishment. But today it is generally accepted as a valid alternative treatment for acute low-back pain.

Palmer believed that the correct alignment of the spinal column is vitally important if good health is to be maintained throughout the body. He felt that if the nerves that connect the brain to the body and its organs became impeded in any way, the flow of nerve impulses to those areas would become sluggish. In turn, he believed, this would result in damage to the tissues and organs supplied by any affected nerve, and, as a consequence, lead to medical disorders affecting areas other than the musculoskeletal system.

Chiropractic theory Palmer believed that inside each person was an "Innate Intelligence"—similar to the concept of "chi" or life-force, which underlies many other alternative therapies—that maintains the body in a state of health. In his theory, any reduction in the flow of nerve impulses, caused most often by a nerve being impeded as it leaves the spinal cord at the spine (page 20), prevents innate intelligence from passing around the body, or reduces the amount that does so. And, according to Palmer's theory, any organ or part of the body that is deprived of sufficient "innate intelligence" is likely to become diseased or will function badly, and symptoms such as pain or stiffness are the result.

Chiropractors call anything that causes the nerves to become impeded a "subluxation," referring to any misalignment or maladjustment of the vertebrae that impinges on spinal nerves as they leave the spinal cord. (In orthodox medicine, the term is used to mean a partial or incomplete dislocation of any two bones at a joint.)

Choosing a practitioner It takes four years to train as a Doctor of Chiropractic (DC) and an undergraduate course is necessary before the training starts. The course does not include surgery or pharmacology, but emphasizes anatomy and physiology, manipulation techniques, and radiology. There are around 70,000 practitioners in the USA.

The American Chiropractic Association (www.acatoday.org), the main representative body, can provide information on practitioners in your area.

Consulting a chiropractor What is likely to happen on your first consultation will depend, in part, on the type of chiropractor you choose. But it is likely that you will be asked about your medical history and lifestyle before being given a physical examination, checking your posture, the curvature of your spine, your reflexes, your range of movement, and the length of your legs. An X-ray of your spine may also be taken and your blood pressure checked.

Treatment normally starts at the second session. The aim is to correct any spinal misalignments, restore a full range of movement, relax and lengthen tense muscles, tendons, and ligaments, correct faulty posture, and to relieve any pain caused by overstimulated nerves. It's sensible to ask for an estimate of how many treatment sessions you are likely to need.

Treatment techniques The principal procedure used by chiropractors is a form of manipulation known as an "adjustment." An adjustment—and there are around 55 of them in a chiropractor's repertoire—consists of a sudden, short, controlled thrust against a joint to extend the range of the joint capsule and surrounding tissues. The speed of the thrust ensures that the muscles have no time to contract and so restrict the movement. A popping sound may be heard during the thrust: this is caused by gases in the synovial fluid (page 17) and is harmless.

Chiropractors also use techniques, such as massage, the application of heat or ice, and kneading, to relax a patient's muscles before a manipulation, to release trigger points (page 187), or to lengthen tendons and muscles. While the vast majority of chiropractic manipulations are safe, if you choose to consult a chiropractor,

IN PRACTICE
A chiropractor will carry out "adjustments," which are rapid thrusts to stretch the joint capsules.

keep in mind that manipulation of the spine, and especially the cervical area carries some risks, particularly to the very young and the very old. Chiropractic manipulations of the neck have been implicated in nerve damage and strokes. Certainly the spine should never be manipulated if there are any signs of nerve involvement, such as a loss of sensation in the legs or impaired bladder control, or if there is bone disease, such as osteoporosis or cancer, a recent fracture, or serious circulatory problems, such as an aneurysm or a history of thrombosis (blood clots).

The Evidence ▸▸

There are well-documented studies that show the beneficial effect of chiropractic treatment for low back pain. For example, research by the well-respected, California-based Rand Corporation shows that chiropractic treatment of back problems—in particular of acute low back pain—generally hastens recovery when compared to more orthodox treatments. But the efficacy of chiropractic as a treatment of problems other than those of the musculoskeletal system remains unproven.

Massage Therapy

Massage relaxes the muscles of the back and eases the tension that contributes to back problems. A deep massage can also break down trigger points—particular areas in most large muscles that tend to go into spasm, forming tight knots that hurt if they are touched or rubbed—so that the muscles function normally and the body regains correct alignment.

Massage therapy has been around for centuries in one form or another, and today it is one of the most popular complementary techniques in America—with an estimated 300,000 practitioners. Classic massage, as practiced by most massage therapists and physical therapists (page 178), uses long, flowing strokes, together with gliding movements, kneading, friction, vibration, and rhythmic tapping. It aims to relax muscles, correct muscle imbalance, stretch tense muscles, and increase flexibility and mobility. And, in the right hands, it succeeds.

Myofascial release "Fascia" (page 19) is connective tissue that surrounds most structures in the body—and especially muscles—to provide support and protection. Unfortunately, like muscles, the fascia can become damaged, whether torn, inflamed, strained by overuse, or weakened by underuse, which causes it to tighten.

Fascial damage limits the free movement of the muscle it encases and can cause stiffness and pain—especially in the back. And the problem can spread to surrounding muscles and structures, so that large areas are affected, resulting in muscular imbalance, poor posture, and back problems.

A massage therapist can detect such taut, inflexible areas by touch and relieve them through myofascial release ("myo" is the Greek word for muscle). The technique is designed to stretch taut fascia in either superficial or deep muscles by using manual stretching and pressure. Working slowly from one area to the next, the therapist eases the tightness and frees the fascia so that the muscles can work to their full potential.

Consulting a practitioner Always check that the massage therapist you choose is properly qualified and accredited by a body such as The National Certification Board for Therapeutic Massage and Bodywork (NCBTMB). In most states it is illegal for massage therapists to practice unless they meet the licensing requirements of that state. You should also check with your local health board, because some towns and cities have further regulations. A list of practitioners may be found at the NCBTMB website (www.ncbtmb.org).

It is also important to check on the nature of the massage offered. Some practitioners offer treatments that are based on belief systems that are not recognized by mainstream medical practitioners. So check with your family physician before you have a massage—especially if any back problem has been diagnosed. Then tell your therapist about any problem you have. Importantly, too: do not allow your therapist to press on your spine or manipulate it in any way.

Trigger Point Therapy ▸▸

Doctors and massage therapists define the term "trigger point" as a small area of muscle fibers that is prone to becoming over-excited and going into spasm. Physicians disagree as to whether trigger points develop as a result of damage, postural problems, and so on, or whether everyone has specific trigger points that are "control centers" for areas of muscle fibers.

Where are they found? These tender spots are often found in the muscles of the back and can be both the result and cause of poor posture. For example, hunching your shoulders means that your neck muscles are perpetually contracted, which over time causes chronic fatigue and strain of the muscle fibers, which go into spasm, creating a painful, tight area. This makes it painful to stretch the muscles fully, so they are always held tight— a vicious circle.

How can massage therapy help? Many massage therapists practice trigger point therapy, as do physical therapists (page 178). It is similar to myofascial release, though muscles are targeted rather than fascia. It aims to release muscle fibers that are in spasm. First the therapist will locate the tender spot (even when pressed gently it can be amazingly painful and you may yelp or jump) and then use slowly increasing pressure to force a degree of relaxation. Once the spot relaxes, the surrounding taut bands of muscle fibers are gently stretched, massaged, and warmed.

The Alexander Technique

The Alexander Technique aims to undo poor, ingrained habits and replace them with the correct, natural movement of early childhood. Young children stand and move with ease and poise, but adults often lose the ability to do this as a result of prolonged sitting, bad lifting techniques, poor posture, pain, and stress.

CAREFUL ADJUSTMENT
An Alexander teacher will carefully and repeatedly adjust your posture so that good posture will eventually feel "right."

Frederick Matthias Alexander, who invented The Alexander Technique, believed that the relationship of the head with the neck and back governs the way the rest of the body functions. He called this relationship the "primary control." If it is balanced and free, the postural muscles (page 149)—the muscles that hold us upright against gravity—work without effort and tension, allowing the phasic muscles—the ones that are activated to make a specific movement—to move the joints freely. If the relationship is faulty, the postural muscles become tense and the phasic muscles have to work harder to achieve a movement. The result is that, over time, the body loses its grace and suppleness. Bad postural habits—known to Alexander teachers as "patterns of misuse"—become ingrained with time, so that the incorrect posture or movement feels "right" and the loss of flexibility and aches and pains are assumed to have another cause.

Teachers of the technique aim to restore the length, coordination, and flexibility of the spine and head—"the primary control"—and re-establish the correct relative position of the two, whether still or in motion.

From the neck down The reason why the head and neck are so easily moved out of their correct position is anatomical. The head rests on a simple, small pivot joint at the top of the spine, but its center of gravity is not in line with the spine. It is much further forward: approximately in the middle of a line drawn between the top of your ear and your cheekbone. Apart from when lying down, our neck muscles are always slightly contracted to pull against the weight and maintain the sensitive balance that keeps the head in its correct position.

The problem is that the neck muscles often become too tense, either for psychological or postural reasons. The result is that the neck muscles pull the head back and down.

The Benefits ►►

The Alexander Technique does not aim to treat specific problems, rather to teach you how to release tension held in muscles caused by habitual poor posture and unnecessary movements and how to relearn correct use.

The benefits claimed include:

■ More freedom of movement.

■ Improved coordination and balance.

■ An increase in energy levels.

■ Improved relaxation.

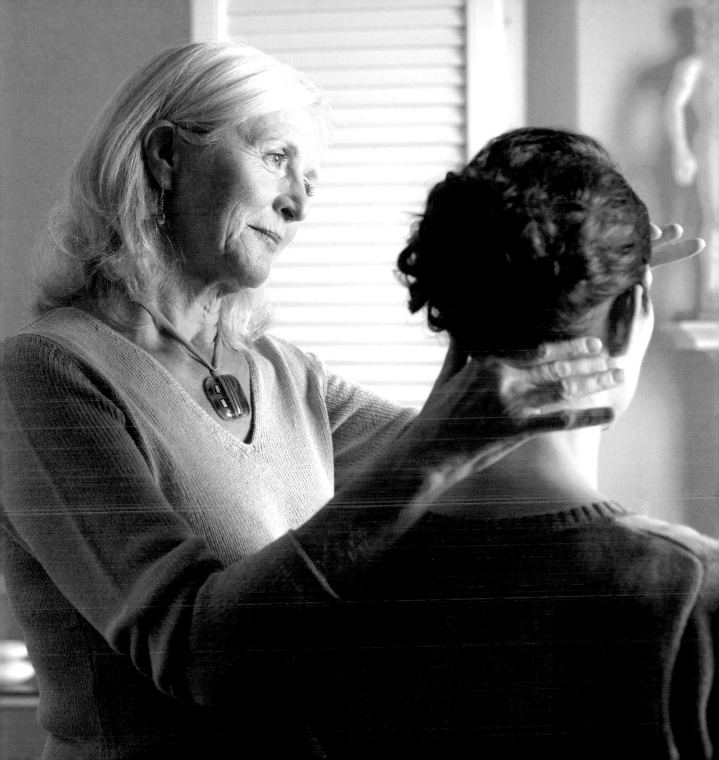

"Good use" in Everyday Life ►►

The Alexander Technique was developed in the late-19th century by Frederick Matthias Alexander (1869–1955). An Australian Shakespearian actor from Tasmania, Alexander found that his voice often became hoarse and croaky. After physicians had failed to find the cause, he noticed that he held his head in an "unnatural way" when talking and walking. After correcting his posture he found that the problem with his voice disappeared. Later, Alexander gave up acting and devoted himself to developing a system that would correct "poor use" habits and promote "good use" posture and movement in everyday life. Three years after Alexander's death in 1955, his followers set up the Society of Teachers of The Alexander Technique (STATS). Today, Alexander teachers worldwide have to complete a three-year training course before they can be registered by STATS.

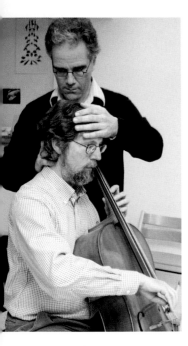

This common postural fault can cause a damaging chain reaction, affecting the postural muscles of the upper, mid, and lower back, compressing the vertebrae and changing the natural alignment of the spine. The result can be problems throughout its length, such as trapped nerves, pain, and restriction of movement. The head's position also inhibits its "primary control" function, which is to initiate and lead any movement.

BOOSTING PERFORMANCE
Alexander Technique is popular among musicians and other performers whose profession involves repetitive movements that can stress the back. Postural adjustment can prevent chronic pain and stiffness.

The three instructions Alexander teachers work according to three main principles, or "instructions," as they call them. It can take considerable time and practice before they become second nature.

To make things easier, Alexander teachers emphasize that you need to "think" every instruction. For example, instead of making a positive movement to take your head up and forward, you should first picture the movement in your mind, which will help your neck muscles to lengthen and relax, and the force of gravity will make the movement occur without any direct command having been sent to the muscles.

- The first and most important instruction is, in Alexander's own words, "to allow the neck to be free"—to relax the muscles of the neck. Most people hold any excess tension whether physical or emotional, in their neck muscles. To see if this applies in your case, rub the muscle running down from your neck and across to your shoulder: if it feels stiff or painful, your neck muscles are over-contracted, short, and tense.
- The second instruction is to lengthen your neck and "allow the head to go forward and upward"— think of the crown of your head rising up and forward, as if you were to nod your head slightly.
- The third of Alexander's instructions was to broaden the back and elongate the whole spinal column. This reduces tension in the muscles of the back and trunk, lengthens the torso, and facilitates abdominal breathing.

Correcting posture the Alexander way Teachers use both their hands and voice commands to help students move correctly from one position to the next, asking them to repeat movements until the students can "feel" the correct position and maintain it. With practice, students become aware of the correct alignment to each other of the head, neck, and back. Specifically, the teacher looks at:

- The angle of your neck and the way in which your neck is supported. The teacher often uses gentle pressure to prevent you from pulling your head back.
- The way in which you move from a sitting to a standing position. It is important to maintain the correct alignment of the neck and spine throughout the movement. The teacher will teach you how to monitor yourself and how to develop awareness of how you make the transition from sitting to standing.
- Your posture in the standing position. The teacher encourages you to adopt a balanced, upright posture before you start to walk.
- Your transition from from standing to walking. The teacher uses his or her hands to prevent your head from dipping forward and your chin from sinking down during movement.

Is It For You? ▸▸

Consult your family physician or internal medicine specialist to check that using The Alexander Technique is appropriate in light of your particular back problems and circumstances. Generally, doctors are very supportive of the technique and its aims. You should also make sure, that your chosen teacher is properly accredited and appropriately insured, for example by checking with the American Society of Alexander Teachers (www.amsatonline.org).

Common Faults ▸▸

The Alexander Technique identifies a number of common faults with posture and movement that can eventually cause back strain and make you more susceptible to injury:

- The whole body is slouched.
- One shoulder is held higher than the other.
- One arm is held farther forward than the other.
- The shoulders are always tense.
- The head pokes forward when walking.
- The knees are braced back rigidly when standing.
- The knees are either allowed to roll out when sitting or are crossed.
- The head is pulled too far back and the back is bent while sitting down.
- When sitting, the feet either do not touch the ground or are bent under the chair with only the toes in contact with the ground.

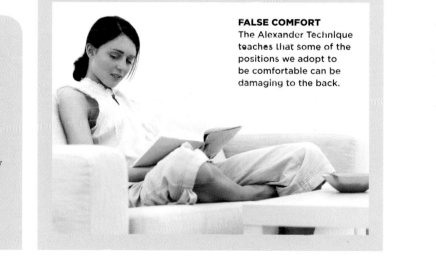

FALSE COMFORT
The Alexander Technique teaches that some of the positions we adopt to be comfortable can be damaging to the back.

The Pilates Method

Pilates is a mind-body exercise therapy that focuses on developing the body's core strength—not just the abdominal muscles but the deep stabilizers of the neck and shoulders, the spine and the pelvis—as well as giving a whole body workout. Its low-impact exercises tone muscles, increase flexibility and control, and improve posture.

Who Was Pilates? ▸▸

The Pilates Method is named after Joseph Hubertus Pilates, its inventor, who was born in Germany in 1880. He was a frail child who suffered from asthma and rickets, and in his battle to overcome these problems he became a gymnast, a circus performer, and an athlete. He developed a mind-body therapy that focused on physical fitness and rehabilitation and called it "Contrology." After his death in 1967, aged 87, "Contrology" was renamed "The Pilates Method."

STRETCH AND STRENGTHEN
Pilates exercises aim to enhance fitness by improving muscle control and flexibility.

The Pilates Method is a very safe form of exercise therapy and is suitable for most people of all ages and fitness levels. It helps prevent neck and back pain and alleviates aches and pains that already exist; and its exercises may help to prevent osteoporosis (page 68). Pilates can also help in conditions such as osteoarthritis (page 58), some spinal curvatures (page 52) and ankylosing spondylosis (page 66). It can offer a safe form of exercise for pregnant and postnatal women (under the guidance of a specially trained Pilates teacher), but you should seek your physician's advice before doing Pilates if you are pregnant.

Core principles The six main principles of the Pilates Method are:

- **Concentration** Each exercise must be performed with full concentration, focusing not only on the movement but the whole body.
- **Control** Each movement must be performed in a precise, accurate, graceful, and controlled manner.
- **Centering** Pilates exercises start by "engaging" (activating) core muscles.
- **Efficiency of movement** Exercises should flow from the core to the extremities (the limbs) and once each exercise is mastered should flow from one exercise to the next.
- **Precision** Each movement must be performed correctly each time with an economy of movement. It is more important to do one exercise correctly than a number of them in a slapdash fashion.
- **Correct, controlled breathing** Pilates teachers believe it is vital to inhale as deeply as possible to increase the oxygen levels in the blood. To help

do this, a forced exhalation empties the lungs of as much air as possible and is followed by deep diaphragmatic inhalation, concentrating on expanding the rib cage.

Pilates and your back Muscular imbalances—for example, if the abdominal muscles are weaker than the back muscles—weak postural muscles generally, a lack of flexibility, and pelvic instability all affect the back adversely. The Pilates Method addresses these problems, increasing core strength by working to create a strong, flexible trunk and pelvic muscles that support and stabilize the spine. This significantly reduces the likelihood of strained muscles and tendons and sprained ligaments as you go about your daily life.

Poor posture is also responsible for many back problems, as it puts pressure on areas of the spine that are not designed to support it, increasing wear and tear and the possibility of inflamed facet joints and damaged disks. Pilates teaches good posture, not just while you are stationary but during movements—through "alignments" as they are called in the Method. Learning correct, symmetrical posture and the correct alignment of the spine—maintaining its natural curvatures—decreases the wear and tear resulting from uneven stresses on the intervertebral joints and disks.

Types of Pilates There are two main schools of Pilates: classical (authentic) and contemporary. Classical Pilates teaches the exercises in an unvarying, strict order that follows Joseph Pilates original ideas closely and uses apparatus based on his designs.

Contemporary Pilates is a modern take on the classical Method in the light of more advanced understanding of body systems. It breaks the Method down into different parts and levels, generally "beginners," "intermediate," and "advanced." A variety of classes are available, ranging from ones held in high-tech studios full of equipment to ones in community centers with just basic mats and exercise balls.

Once you are familiar with the principles and the exercises you can practice at home with the help of the numerous books and DVDs that are available. And why not try out the basic Pilates lower back exercises shown on the following pages?

Who Can Teach Pilates? ⏩

In 2000 a U.S. Federal court ruled that "Pilates" was a generic term and could be used without restriction. As a result, anyone can offer "Pilates" to the general public—whether properly trained in the Pilates method or not.

In response, associations to register properly trained teachers of the Pilates Method were set up in a number of countries. In the US, one such body providing accreditation and certification is called The Pilates Method Alliance (www.pilatesmethodalliance. org). Before you enroll in a Pilates class, it is sensible to check the teacher's accreditation and to make sure that he or she has appropriate insurance cover.

How to start The best way to introduce yourself to Pilates is to join a class run by an accredited, insured teacher. The beginner's series of Pilates exercises is the most beneficial for people who are suffering from back problems.

If you suffer from any medical condition check with your doctor before starting a Pilates class. Tell your teacher about any problems that you have, too, so that exercises can be adapted to suit your needs. And if you are seeing a physical therapist for rehabilitation purposes, ask him or her to outline your rehabilitation priorities and goals to your Pilates teacher.

These exercises help correct imbalances in the muscles of the lower back by stretching and improving the tone of weaker muscles. The Pilates philosophy emphasizes the importance of engaging both body and mind, so concentrate fully on what you are doing and make precise, controlled, slow movements. Repeat each exercise up to five times. One caveat: don't attempt these exercises if you have any pre-existing condition—including brachialgia (page 116) or sciatica (page 118)—unless advised to do so by your physician or physical therapist, and observe the cautions on page 10.

Forward stretch
Increases the lower back's range of movement.

1 Sit up straight, keeping your spine's natural curves, with your legs straight. Place your feet shoulder-width apart with the toes pointing toward the ceiling. Lift your arms to shoulder height.

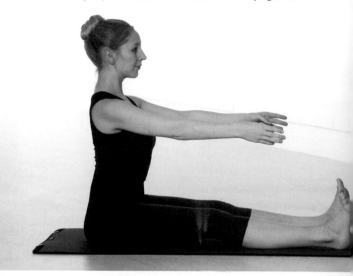

2 Inhale. Then, while exhaling slowly and drawing in your abdominal muscles, roll your head back and forward to form a U-shape. Hold for a count of five. Inhale, then exhale slowly and return to the starting position. Repeat five times.

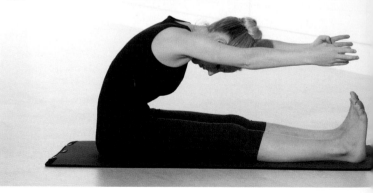

Hamstring stretch

Releases tension in the lower back.

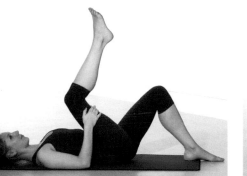 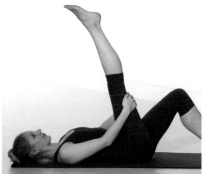 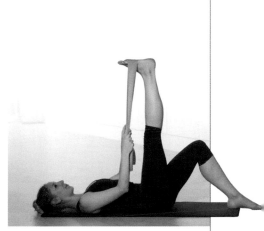

1 Lie on your back with your knees bent at 90 degrees and your feet shoulder-width apart. Raise your left leg, supporting the thigh with your hands if necessary.

2 Inhale, then, while exhaling slowly and drawing in your abdominal muscles, raise your leg vertically. Hold for a count of five, then repeat with your other leg. Repeat five times.

Alternative You may find it more comfortable to use a belt or exercise band around the foot to raise your leg toward the ceiling. Try both methods to see which you prefer.

The arrow

Strengthens lower back muscles.

1 Lie face down. (Rest your head on a folded towel if you find this more comfortable.) Place your arms by your sides with the palms facing upward.

2 Inhale. Then, while exhaling slowly and drawing in your abdominal muscles, raise your arms to the horizontal and lift your head, chest, and shoulders slightly— keep your neck and back in a straight line Hold for a count of five.

3 Inhale as you slowly lower your arms, neck, and back to the starting position. Repeat five times.

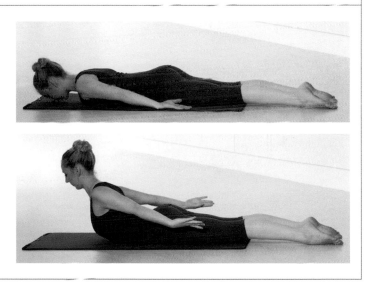

Yoga

In 2010, according to statistics published by the *Yoga Journal,* 14.3 million Americans had practiced yoga in that year, compared with 4.3 million in 2004. And other studies have shown that the majority of those who have taken up the practice had been recommended to do so by their doctor. It's clear that yoga has become a treatment of choice for many.

Yoga has been around for at least 5,000 years, but has only become popular in the West relatively recently. Its attractions are twofold: it is an effective form of exercise that develops flexibility, stretches and strengthens the muscles, and mobilizes the joints; it also relaxes the mind. All of which makes it ideal for the prevention of many back problems and the treatment of some of them, including poor posture, chronic back pain, osteoarthritis (page 58), and—some recent studies indicate—rheumatoid arthritis (page 62).

There are numerous different yoga systems, which stress spirituality to different degrees. It is important, though, to be clear that the physical exercises of yoga have nothing to do with religion and do not clash with any religious tradition. The most popular form is hatha yoga, which combines poses (asanas), physical movements, and breathing techniques. The latter aim to fill and empty the lungs fully, using rhythmic inhalations and exhalations controlled by the diaphragm. Achieving a balance between strength and flexibility in the back muscles is also stressed.

The only drawback is that yoga is a technique that should be taught first and then practiced regularly to achieve its full benefits. After attending classes, you can put what you have learned into practice at home, but you will be expected to develop further by maintaining your relationship with your teacher. A number of yoga poses and movements are very good for increasing spinal flexibility and strength to prevent back problems from arising, but, again, it is far better—and safer—if you are taught how to carry them out by a qualified yoga teacher.

Does it work? Anecdotally, yes, it does work. There have also been a number of small-scale research studies in America on the effectiveness of yoga in the prevention of chronic back pain and its relief. The results have been promising, but they cannot be said to amount to scientific proof. A recent study conducted by the University of York in the U.K. found that those with back pain who practiced yoga in addition to conventional medical treatment experienced greater improvements than those who received only standard care.

Is it safe? While yoga is safe for most people, it is sensible to take certain precautions. Do not practice yoga if you are pregnant, because some of the poses may endanger your pregnancy—it's fine to continue with your breathing exercises, though, and to meditate if that's part of your yoga practice. Some teachers specialize in prenatal yoga, and can advise on safe forms of practice.

Similarly, children should not practice yoga, because their bodies are not sufficiently developed to cope with the stresses and strains of some poses, and, yoga adherents say, their natural growth may be affected—again, breathing techniques are fine.

You should always consult your family physician before starting yoga if you have an existing back problem, because some poses might make it worse—sometimes dangerously so. If you get your doctor's go-ahead, tell your yoga teacher exactly what your problem is. According to the U.S. Consumer Product Safety Commission, there were more than 5,500 yoga-related injuries treated in doctors' offices, clinics, and emergency rooms in 2007. And The American Academy of Orthopaedic Surgeons (AAOS) says of yoga: "the seemingly harmless activities can cause muscle strain, torn ligaments, or more serious injuries if practiced incorrectly . . . [the AAOS] believes the rewards of basic yoga outweigh the potential physical risks, as long as you take caution and perform the exercises in moderation, according to your individual flexibility level." Which makes it vital that you are taught by an experienced, qualified teacher.

Consulting a teacher The main supervisory body is The Yoga Alliance, through whose website (www.yogaalliance.org) you can find a teacher near you. Another body is The American Yoga Association (www.americanyogaassociation.org). And in some areas you may be lucky enough to find a class that specializes in teaching yoga for back problems.

You also need to think about what style of yoga you prefer. Are you more interested in the spiritual aspects rather than the physical benefits? Is so, you may prefer to try out some of the more esoteric types rather than hatha yoga, which focuses on exercises and breathing.

CHILD POSE
This simple stretch is one of the many yoga poses that can help to relieve back pain.

Acupuncture

For thousands of years, Chinese and Japanese physicians relied on acupuncture for maintaining good health and curing disease. The technique has grown increasingly popular in the West and although many doctors dismiss it as quackery, most research seems to support the idea that acupuncture can be effective in treating back problems.

Acupuncture was first heard of by many Americans from accounts that a reporter, James Reston, who accompanied President Nixon on his ground-breaking 1972 visit to China, had been operated on under acupuncture anesthesia. In fact, he had been anesthetized conventionally, and just received acupuncture to ease post-operative cramps. But the original reports took wings, and nowadays, acupuncture is almost a mainstream therapy.

How do people think it works? A key component of traditional Chinese medicine, acupuncture was first described in the 2nd century BCE. At that time, stone and bone needles—they're made of stainless steel wires now—were used to probe a series of points ("acupoints") distributed around the body. These acupoints are located on theoretical energy channels in the body, called "meridians," through which the life force "chi," or "qi," flows. The theory is that disease results from a disruption in the normal flow of chi. The presence of the needles in an acupoint is said to redistribute and normalize the flow of chi and therefore cure or alleviate disease.

Many people are very attracted to ancient therapies, which they see as more "natural" than current Western drug-based or surgical approaches. But there is still no hard evidence that there is any such thing as chi or, indeed, acupoints. Having said that, there do appear to be trigger points (page 189), that show certain affinities to acupoints and are said to have distinct electrical properties, but they are rarely in the same physical position as traditional acupoints are said to be located.

And does it work? Confusingly, yes and no. Many medical scientists believe that acupuncture can be effective for the relief of pain, but not for the treatment of disease. The American College of Physicians and The American Pain Society concluded in 2008 that clinicians should consider acupuncture among and alongside a range of other, more conventional techniques. Although some physicians and physical therapists practice acupuncture, many do not acknowledge it as an effective therapy.

And it's worth remembering that acupuncture is not risk free. In a German study of nearly 300,000 patients, 8.6 percent reported adverse effects, such as bleeding and bruising; damage has also been caused by acupuncturists needling too close to, or even into, the kidneys. What's more, many patients find acupuncture extremely painful. The bottom line? If you believe that acupuncture holds the hope of resolving your back problem and you have found a qualified, experienced practitioner in whom you have confidence, you may be in luck.

Choosing a practitioner Laws on whether acupuncturists can treat you with or without medical supervision vary from state to state—check out The Home of Traditional Chinese Medicine website to see what rules apply to you (www. acupuncture.com). And you can use www.nccaom. org to find a licensed acupuncturist (L.AC) or a Diplomate of Acupuncture (Dipl. Ac).

It is also sensible to check with your medical insurers before you book a course of treatment: many will pay for it, depending on what's wrong, but others will not.

Alternatively, you could choose to consult a medical doctor who practices acupuncture—look at the American Academy of Medical Acupuncture website for details (www.medicalacupuncture.org).

What happens during a consultation? What your acupuncturist will do at a consultation depends on his or her belief system. Followers of traditional acupuncture, and traditional Chinese medicine are likely to look closely at your face and tongue, listen to your breathing, assess your body odor, ask about your general health and bodily functions, check your body for tender points, and also feel 12 pulses on your arms.

Medical acupuncturists, are less likely to follow this approach. Instead, having made a diagnosis on conventional grounds, they are likely to use acupuncture primarily to relieve pain.

A word of caution If you do visit an acupuncturist, make sure that he or she uses sterile needles, preferably disposable ones, so that you are treated with a brand new set at every visit. Re-used, unsterile needles can lead to potentially life-threatening infections.

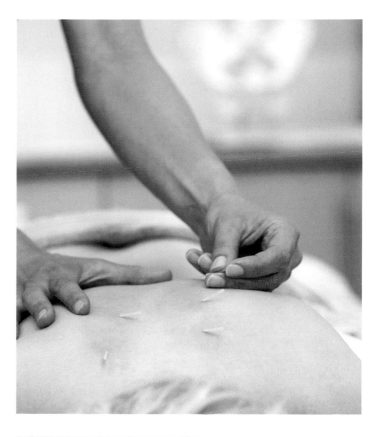

Skip the Herbs ▸▸

Some practitioners prescribe herbs as well as acupuncture: do not take these until you have discussed them with your family physician, because they are usually chemically active and may interfere with the action of other medications.

NEEDLING THE PAIN
When you have acupuncture treatment, following an assessment of your symptoms, the practitioner will insert very fine needles into the acupoints he or she judges to be of most benefit in your case.

Shiatsu

Derived from the ancient Chinese therapeutic massage system called *anmo*, modern shiatsu (*shi* means "fingers" and *atsu* means "pressure") was developed in Japan by Tamai Tempaku in 1919. It may be based on traditional techniques, but it is one of the most modern of the therapies that rely on the flow of our "life force."

Tempaku's new shiatsu combined anmo with concepts of the life force ki, the Japanese form of chi (page 198). Later, three of his students developed different forms of shiatsu, which are the ones most often offered in the West: "Zen shiatsu," "Namikosho shiatsu," and "acupressure shiatsu."

Zen shiatsu is the form most widely practiced in the West. It relies on a complex diagnostic system but uses largely the same acupoints (page 198) as acupuncture and the same meridians, and aims to restore ki to normality.

Namikosho shiatsu is less concerned with ki and meridians, relying on the rubbing and pressing techniques of anmo. It also takes Western ideas of anatomy, physiology, and neurology into account.

Acupressure shiatsu, the last of the three forms, falls somewhere between the other two systems. Also called "tsubo therapy"—tsubo is the Japanese word for an acupoint—it concentrates on stimulating the relevant tsubos by means of massage, non-penetrating needles, electrical devices, and the application of heat.

Many shiatsu practitioners also use healing techniques, such as visualizing the transmission of healing energy into the patient's body, techniques derived from Western physical therapy, such as passive rotations and stretches, and general body massage.

Does it work? It may, but there is little scientific evidence to show that it does—a large-scale review of the available evidence in 2007, commissioned by the Shiatsu Society U.K., concluded that "there was insufficient evidence both in quantity and quality on shiatsu." Nor is there any convincing evidence, in terms of Western science, that ki, meridians, and tsubos physically exist. But many people have reported an improvement in symptoms caused by muscle and joint problems after a shiatsu treatment session and feelings of stress-free relaxation.

In general, shiatsu is very safe when performed by a trained shiatsuist but check with your doctor before visiting one if you are receiving any form of medical treatment. Do not have shiatsu treatment during pregnancy, since stimulation of certain areas can affect the womb.

Finding a practitioner The shiatsu practitioner you choose depends largely on which system you find the most attractive. There are also a large number of sub-systems, each of which has its own diagnostic and treatment practices. So check what system your practitioner uses and ask for details of what type of diagnosis and treatment is on offer before you make your choice. Different states have different laws about the practice of shiatsu—as do many cities and counties. Many of them require a practitioner to be certified in massage therapy, which is highly regulated. Generally this is certified by The National Certification Board for Therapeutic Massage and Bodywork (NCBTMB), and you can find a practitioner on its website (www.ncbtmb.org). The only way to find out what laws apply in your area is to contact your local health board.

Shiatsu's governing body is The American Organization for Bodywork Therapies of Asia (AOBTA). It has a *Find a Practitioner* page on its website (www.aobta.org).

Diagnosis and treatment The information on these pages refers primarily to Zen shiatsu, since it is the most common form of the therapy. Clothes are worn throughout a session—ideally you should wear loose-fitting, light garments. You will usually receive treatment on the floor, lying on a futon or a thin mattress.

First, the practitioner will diagnose the overall state of your ki, take your medical history, and then make general observations through hearing, smelling, and visual clues.

But a practitioner's most important diagnostic tool is touch. Shiatsuists believe that several areas of the body form a map of the whole body, and that information about the state of ki in a particular organ can be gained by palpating the part of the map that relates to it.

In the context of back problems, the most important map is of "yu" points (also known as back transporting points") alongside the spine, though the "hara" map of the abdomen is also important. The relative tenderness, softness, or hardness of the points in the relevant map is revealed by palpation, and gives the shitasuist information about the energy balance in different structures and organs. Wrist pulses may also be

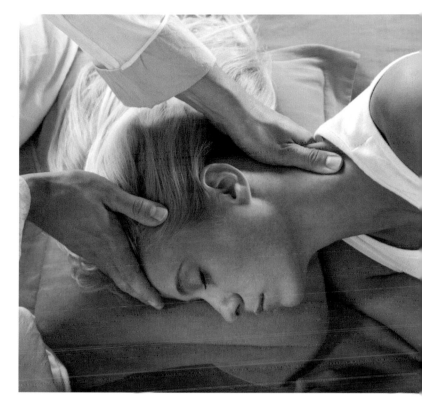

taken—there are different positions for each meridian. Treatment then starts, though diagnosis continues throughout the process as your responses to it are observed.

Meridians are massaged using a variety of techniques, but there may also be more general muscle and joint mobilizations and stretches involving the whole body—not dissimilar to those used in physical therapy (page 178)—as well as deep pressure techniques. Throughout, the shiatsuist will try to transmit healing energy to you and stimulate the your own self-healing capacity.

DIAGNOSTIC TOUCH
A shiatsu practitioner will first use touch to diagnose your problem in terms of shiatsu theory, and then will use pressure, massage, and manipulations to treat it.

TENS

Since its introduction some 30 years ago, TENS—transcutaneous electrical nerve stimulation—has become a popular self-help treatment, especially for back pain. Although it is only intended to reduce pain rather than to address the cause of the pain, the relief of pain can sometimes help to resolve problems such as muscles spasms and imbalances.

TENS uses electrical current to stimulate nerves. It should not be confused with EMS (electrical muscle stimulation), which, as the name suggests, is designed to stimulate muscle activity, although sometimes both TENS functions and EMS are combined in the same machine.

The underlying theory TENS relies on the "gate theory of pain" first proposed in 1965. This has never been conclusively proved, but is nevertheless viewed as convincing by most scientists.

Here's how it may work: The sensation of pain is transmitted to the brain in two different ways. Sudden onset pain is transmitted by fast, large-diameter, myelin-insulated "A-fiber" nerves, at about 30 feet (9 m) per second; chronic pain is transmitted by slower, small-diameter, uninsulated "C-fiber" nerves at about 3 feet (90 cm) per second. Pain receptors work on an all or nothing system. When they are stimulated beyond a certain threshold, they send a message of pain to the brain; if the stimulation fails to reach the threshold, no signal is sent.

Pain varies in intensity not because the signals are stronger or weaker but because of differences in the number and frequency of messages the brain receives. And even when a pain signal has been sent, it may not reach the brain. That's because there are three junctions, or "gates," between the pain receptors and the brain.

The first junction is in the spinal cord, and this gate can only take a limited amount of traffic. If too many signals try to get through the gate, priority is given to the fast A-fibers: signals traveling along the slower C-fibers simply cannot get through.

Once the first flood of sudden onset pain impulses has died down, the messages carried by the C-fibers are allowed to pass through again. The spinal cord also contains nerve pathways that can close the gate and eliminate all pain. This is the survival mechanism that sometimes allows a soldier to fight on even when severely wounded.

The other pain gates, which are located in the brain, operate on a different principle. These gates use the body's own natural painkillers, chemicals called endorphins, to reduce or block the reception of pain signals in the brain.

How it works TENS works by stimulating the C-fibers to such an extent that the A-fibers responding to acute pain are blocked out; it may also increase the activity of the inhibitory nerve at the spinal gate; and, at low frequency, may increase the production of endorphins, the body's own natural painkiller in the brain.

How to use TENS It is difficult to generalize about using TENS, because machines from different manufacturers have different controls and carry different recommendations.

What all TENS machines have in common is the use of two electrodes, normally hidden inside pads. One should be placed on the muscle closest to the pain. The second electrode should be placed closer to your spine than the first, but not directly over it, if the pain is in your back, shoulder, or hip. The electrodes should not touch.

Start by using TENS for about 20 minutes, about three to four times a day. When you are used to this, you can build up to 30 minutes at a time as often as you like, but you should take regular breaks. Don't use it in bed at night.

The Evidence ▸▸

Surprisingly for such a popular treatment, there is little hard evidence—as opposed to anecdotal accounts—that TENS has a measurable effect on back pain. For example, in 2007 the Cochrane Collaboration, a prestigious international research body, stated, "At this time, the evidence reported from a small number of placebo-controlled trials does not support the use of TENS in the routine management of low-back pain."

Of course, this does not mean that TENS is always ineffective—merely that it has not been conclusively proved to work in the majority of cases. And since many thousands of people testify to the benefits of TENS—whether because thinking that it works has beneficial effects or because it does, in fact, have a therapeutic effect—it may be sensible to try. The decision is yours.

Sensible precautions TENS should always be used with care and according to the manufacturer's instructions. Do not, for example, use TENS:

- On broken skin.
- On your skull.
- Anywhere near your eyes.
- Near your mouth.
- On the front or sides of your neck.
- Internally.
- In the area of a tumor.
- From front to back of the chest or vice versa.
- On children.
- When sleeping.

In the following cases, you should not use a TENS machine without checking with your family physician because to do so could be dangerous:

- You're pregnant.
- You suffer from epilepsy.
- You have heart disease.
- You have a pacemaker.
- Your pain is of unknown cause.

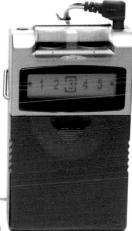
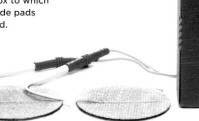

TENS MACHINE
The equipment for administering TENS typically consists of a control box to which two electrode pads are attached.

Drug Treatment

A huge number of drugs treatments are used to treat back problems, either prescribed by your doctor or bought over-the-counter (OTC) without a prescription at your local pharmacy. But whether on prescription or not, many of them can have serious side effects and some are highly addictive. Take them only on your doctor's advice.

On the following pages you'll find descriptions of the principal medications used in the treatment of back problems. They are grouped according to their main action or use along with the descriptions of specific generic drugs (common brand names are in italic type).

As each individual's medical history is different and some medicines and herbal remedies react with each other, these pages are only a guide to what OTC medicines might help and the drugs that your medical practitioner might prescribe. If you are already taking any medicines it is important to check with your doctor before using OTC products; remember, too, to check the medication's accompanying instructional leaflet and its dosage advice before you take it.

Also be aware that some OTC medicines have more than one active ingredient—for example, acetaminophen is combined with other ingredients in a number of them, which means that if you are not careful you could take too much of it if you are also using other medications. Always check the label to see what active ingredients the medication contains. And do not take alcohol with them. A woman should always tell her physician or pharmacist if there is any possibility that she may be pregnant.

PAINKILLERS

Acetaminophen (*Panadol, Tylenol*) This widely used OTC painkiller, usually considered in a class of its own, is often used to relieve pain caused by general back problems and muscle and joint problems; preparations are available that are

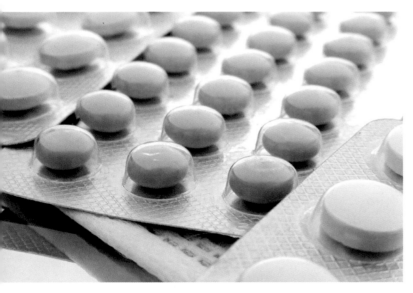

KNOW YOUR MEDICINES
Help yourself to be more actively involved in your recovery by informing yourself about the medicines prescribed for you.

Smooth Away Pain ▸▸

Skin creams that contain the active ingredient in chili peppers, capsaicin (for example, *Capsagel*, *Zotrix*) and those that contain methylsalicylate/menthol (*BenGay*, *Icy Hot*) are commonly used to relieve back pain. The former work by interfering with action of a chemical called "substance P," which helps transmit pain signals to the brain. Research has shown that such creams are effective, but may take a week or two before they reduce your pain. The latter type have a more immediate impact: they first cool and then heat the skin and underlying tissues, distracting you from feeling pain.

Allergic reactions to these creams are rare but do occur, so consult your physician immediately if you experience any adverse effects. And make sure that you never use these skin creams over broken skin or allow them to come into contact with your eyes.

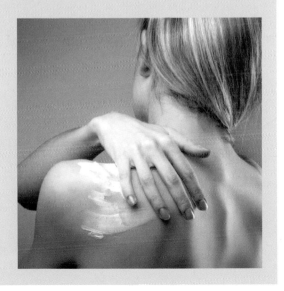

suitable for children. You need to stick rigidly to the dose recommendation made by your doctor because overdose can cause serious liver damage.

NSAIDs (nonsteroidal anti-inflammatory drugs) These work by blocking the production of prostaglandins, chemicals that are produced as a response to damage or injury and cause pain, swelling, inflammation, and fever. Prostaglandins also sensitize nerve endings and so increase your perception of pain. NSAIDS are both painkillers and anti-inflammatories, and are used to treat general aches and pains—such as headaches, muscle strains, ligament sprains, and painful joints—as well as osteoarthritis (page 58), rheumatoid arthritis (page 62), and ankylosing spondylitis (page 66). The commonest side effects are stomach upsets and bleeding in the digestive tract.

Always take these drugs with food to avoid stomach upsets, although bleeding remains a risk. You should not take NSAIDs if you are on medication, such as warfarin, to control blood clotting. They should be used with caution by anyone with a history of heart or circulatory problems. And drugs in this group should be avoided during pregnancy

- **Aspirin** Used primarily as a painkiller, it also reduces inflammation and swelling. If you are on a daily dose of aspirin for reducing cardiovascular risk it is better not to take any other NSAID. Some people are allergic to aspirin and need to be aware of multi-ingredient products that contain it. Aspirin can also cause stomach problems, such as bleeding and ulcers. And anyone under 19 should never be given aspirin (or any medicine that contains aspirin), because of the risk of triggering Reye's syndrome, a potentially fatal condition.

- **Ibuprofen** (*Motrin, Advil*) For muscle and joint problems, backache, and general aches and pains, as well as inflammatory diseases such as rheumatoid arthritis.
- **Naproxen** (*Aleve*) Used in particular to treat osteoarthritis, rheumatoid arthritis, ankylosing spondylitis, and musculoskeletal problems.
- **Diclofenac** One of the strongest NSAIDs, it is long-lasting and sometimes need only be taken once a day. It is especially useful in the treatment of chronic pain, as in osteoarthritis, rheumatoid arthritis, and ankylosing spondylitis. As with all NSAIDs, there is a risk of stomach upsets and bleeds. Diclofenac is also available in topical form that can be applied directly to the affected area.
- **Celecoxib** (*Celebrex*) One of the newer NSAIDs known as COX-2 selective inhibitors, it is an advance on other NSAIDs as it carries a lower risk of bleeding in the stomach.

Opiates These drugs, derived from opium, are used to relieve moderate to severe pain. They provide quick pain relief by preventing pain messages from reaching the brain. Opiates also affect the part of the brain that controls pleasure, resulting in feelings of euphoria or a sense of wellbeing. This makes them liable to abuse and they are potentially addictive in the long term. Always stick to the prescribed dosage and never combine them with alcohol. The most common side effect of opiate medications are stomach upset and constipation.

- **Codeine** (*Codeine systemic*) The most widely used opiate, it relieves pain and is mildly sedative. Codeine is also combined with acetaminophen in preparations such as *Tylenol#3* and *#4*.
- **Hydrocodone** (*Lorcet, Vicodin*) This highly addictive semi-synthetic opiate is derived from codeine or thebaine, an opium derivative, and is often combined with acetaminophen.
- **Oxycodone** (*Oxycontin, Percocet, Percodan*) A slow-release opiate derived from thebaine that is often combined with acetaminophen. In long-term use it carries a high risk of addiction.
- **Tramadol** (*Ultram*) For moderate to severe pain, this drug is not an opiate, but works in a similar way. Less addictive than true opiates, it can nevertheless cause addiction in long-term use.

MUSCLE RELAXANTS

As well as helping muscles to relax, these drugs affect the brain to provide overall sedation. The most common medications in this group are:

- **Carisoprodol** (*Soma*) For the short-term relief of moderate to severe back and neck pain caused by muscle spasm.
- **Cylobenzaprine** (*Flexeril*) For moderate to severe muscle spasm; to be taken only for a few weeks.
- **Diazepam** (*Valium*) For moderate to severe muscle spasm. It can also act as a depressant,

so it should be avoided if you have a history of depression. Neither should you take it with alcohol, which can increase its effect. Diazepam is addictive and should be taken for no longer than two weeks.

- **Metaxolone** (*Skelaxin*) For the relief of painful muscle spasm; it is used with analgesics and physical therapy. Avoid alcohol and the herb St. John's wort while taking this drug.

ANTI-INFLAMMATORY DRUGS

This group of drugs that counter inflammation (redness and swelling of body tissues) includes two distinct subgroups, nonsteroidal anti-inflammatory drugs (NSAIDs) and corticosteroids.

NSAIDs Used also for their painkilling effect (see page 205), these drugs reduce inflammation in diseases such as osteoarthritis, rheumatoid arthritis, and ankylosing spondylitis. (For examples of specific drugs, see opposite.)

Corticosteroids Given by mouth, these powerful anti-inflammatory drugs can be useful for severe low-back pain or nerve root problems. They are usually given in a week or two-week course. Long-term use can produce unwanted effects, including osteoporosis, weight gain, and peptic ulcers.

- **Methylprednisolone** This corticosteroid is usually prescribed for rheumatoid arthritis only within two years of diagnosis.

DMARDS

"Disease-modifying antirheumatic drugs" (DMARDs) are a group of medicines that work by curbing the underlying processes that cause rheumatoid arthritis, ankylosing spondylitis, and other inflammatory types of arthritis. They help to minimize the symptoms and also slow degeneration of the joints.

- **Methotrexate** (*Rheumatrex*) The most common and effective first line of treatment for active and severe rheumatoid arthritis and other similar diseases. Unfortunately, methotrexate has many serious side effects, notably on liver function. For this reason, you should only take it after a frank discussion with your physician and also exactly as prescribed. Regular blood tests are usually required during treatment with this drug.
- **Sulfasalazine** (*Azulfidine*) This medicine is approved by the FDA to treat rheumatoid arthritis but can also be used to treat ankylosing spondylitis, if your physician judges it to be of potential benefit. Side effects may include nausea and vomiting, loss of appetite, headache, and rashes. Your urine may also turn orange, though this is harmless. It can also lead to folic acid deficiency and increase the unwanted effects of methotrexate (see above).
- **Hydroxychloroquine** (*Plaquenil*) Antimalarial drugs such as hydroxychloroquine were found to be effective in the treatment of rheumatoid arthritis after patients taking the medication to fight malaria reported improvement in their joint function. These drugs are thought to affect the immune system, but it is not known how or why they improve rheumatoid conditions. This drug can lower your white blood cell count, so you may need regular blood tests.
- **Leflunomide** (*Arava*) This drug helps calm the inflammation associated with rheumatoid arthritis by interfering with cells that cause inflammation and so reduces joint damage, pain, and stiffness. Regular blood and liver function tests are needed

during treatment. Unfortunately, it can also cause birth defects when taken by either parent, so should not be used it you are planning a family.

- **Sodium aurothiomalate** This gold-based preparation acts by reducing inflammation in the joints, though how is not known. It can be given by injection to treat rheumatoid arthritis (page 62)—the most effective way—or if this is not possible, in tablet form.

Tumor necrosis factor blockers (TNFs) This new type of drug has been used since 1998 to treat rheumatoid arthritis and similar conditions. These "biologic" drugs copy substances made naturally by the body's immune system to reduce inflammation. Such drugs are used in cases of moderate to severe rheumatoid arthritis in which DMARDs have not been effective, although they may be used in conjunction with them. These drugs are usually self-administered by injection into the thigh or abdomen. Their main risk is an increased susceptibility to all types of infection, especially tuberculosis. Drugs in this group include adalimumab (*Humira*), anakinra (*Kineret*), and etanercept (*Enbrel*).

NEUROPATHICS
These drugs treat nerve pain, such as sciatica (page 118) in the leg, and brachialgia (page 82) in the arm. Unfortunately, finding the correct drug or combination of drugs to treat nerve pain is often a matter of trial and error.

Tricyclic antidepressants Drugs such as amitriptyline (*Elavil*) are thought to reduce nerve pain by increasing the activity of neurotransmitters in the spinal cord that cut pain signals. It may take several weeks for pain to be relieved by these drugs.

Anticonvulsant medications Some of these drugs (gabapentin/*Neurontin* and pregabalin/*Lyrica*) also used to control seizures, can be highly effective in the relief of nerve pain. Gabapentin can cause suicidal thoughts. So alert people around you and notify your physician immediately if you feel depressed or have any suicidal thoughts. Also be aware that stopping the drug suddenly can lead to seizures.

BONE-DENSITY BUILDERS
In this group are a variety of types of drugs used to improve bone density and strength in those affected by osteoporosis and similar conditions. Many of these medicines affect the action of estrogen, a female sex hormone, which protects bone mass, but also has undesirable effects, such as promoting various types of cancer.

SERMs (selective estrogen receptor modulators) This is a relatively new group of medications that affect estrogen receptors. So far, two drugs in this group have been approved by the Federal Drug Administration (FDA) but others are in the pipeline.

- **Tamoxifen** The best known and oldest SERM, it is primarily used to treat breast cancer but has some beneficial effects on bone mass.
- **Raloxifene** Used to treat osteoporosis in postmenopausal women and some men, this drug reduces the amount of bone that is lost by around 35 percent and increases bone mass density by some 3 percent in the vertebrae. This reduces the incidence of vertebral fractures by between 40 and 50 percent while not encouraging breast cancer or heart problems. Treatment with this drug carries an increased risk of stroke.

Rank ligand inhibitor One of the TNF family of drugs (see left), this medication has a particularly beneficial effect on bone density.

- **Denosumab** (*Prolia, Xgeva*) This drug is given in six monthly injections to postmenopausal women who have not responded to other osteoporosis medications. It works by reducing bone breakdown and increasing bone strength and density. Possible side effects of treatment include rashes, joint pain, tingling of your fingers and toes, and muscle spasms.

Hormone therapy (HT) This treatment for menopausal symptoms, in which supplements of the female sex hormones estrogen and progestogen are given, can also slow bone loss and is therefore of added benefit for menopausal women at risk of osteoporosis. However, HT increases the risk of breast cancer, stroke, and blood clots, so should be used only for limited periods. Discuss the duration of treatment with your physician.

DRUGS THAT AFFECT BONE METABOLISM

Drugs within this category regulate the reabsorption of bone and maintain calcium balance, and so increase bone density.

Biophosphonates Alendronate (*Fosamax*) and risedronate (*Actonel*) can reduce the risk of vertebral, hip, and wrist fractures by between 40 and 50 percent by reducing the effect of cells that break down bone. Although these medications can cause nausea and stomach irritation, there are usually few side effects. Long-term use may be associated with fractures of the femur (thigh bone) and can cause serious jaw problems.

Calcitonin (*Miacalcin*) This drug produces only a small reduction in the risk of vertebral fractures. It is not widely prescribed, because it can cause stomach problems and hot flashes. But it can relieve the pain of a bone fracture.

Parathyroid hormone (PTH) Treatment with a synthetic version of this hormone stimulates bone growth rather than preventing further bone loss, and can deliver up to a 5 percent increase in bone mass density. It reduces the risk of vertebral fracture by as much as 65 percent.

- **Teriparatide** (*Forteo*) This synthetic hormone is given by injection for the treatment of osteoporosis in men and postmenopausal women who are at high risk of suffering a fracture. Possible side effects include heart problems, pain, headaches, nausea, and insomnia.

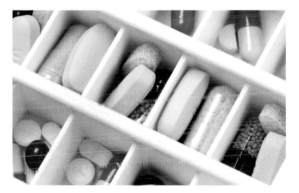

GET ORGANIZED
If your condition requires treatment with multiple medications or if you are sometimes a little forgetful, a handy pill organizer box that has separate compartments for each day can be a great help for preventing missed or repeated doses.

Surgery

Sometimes surgery is used to help resolve back problems. A range of techniques is available, including spinal fusion (which welds vertebrae together), spinal decompression surgery (which reduces pressure on the spinal cord and nerves), and even the replacement of a spinal disk with an artificial one.

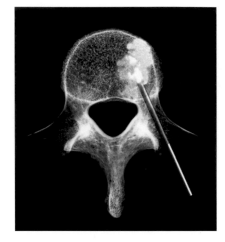

VERTEBROPLASTY IN ACTION
This CT image shows bone-strengthening "cement" being injected into a vertebra affected by osteoporosis.

Whatever surgical option you are considering, it is important to remember that, because of the risks and expense, surgery is generally used only when other, non-invasive treatments have failed or are inappropriate (for example, in the case of a tumor). In addition, surgery is normally only an option when a distinct anatomical problem has been diagnosed by imaging techniques.

Spinal surgery can be difficult to understand because of the large number of highly technical terms that surgeons use to describe their various procedures. On these pages you will find definitions of the more common ones, together with a description of what they entail. Many of the surgical techniques described aim to reduce pressure on the spinal cord and nerve roots (pages 82 and 116). Such pressure causes symptoms such as pain, numbness, weakness, and reduced mobility.

The procedure that your surgeon recommends depends on what part of a vertebra (or vertebrae) is impinging on nerve tissue—either the spinal cord or the nerves that leave it to run to other parts of the body—as well as your general health and the precise nature of your condition.

Injection techniques There are two types of injection technique currently practiced in the U.S.A.: vertebroplasty and kyphoplasty. Both are used for spinal stabilization. These are the least invasive of all the surgical options for back problems.

- **Vertebroplasty** Used to treat compression fractures of vertebrae, which are often caused by osteoporosis (page 68). In it a cement-like mixture is injected into the fractured bone, guided by imaging techniques.
- **Kyphoplasty** A variant of vertebroplasty, in which a tiny balloon is injected into the fractured bone by means of a needle to create a cavity. The balloon is then withdrawn and a cement-like material is injected into the cavity. This procedure can sometimes restore some of the vertebra's original height.

ENDOSCOPIC DISKECTOMY
In this type of minimally invasive surgery for a herniated intervertebral disk, the surgeon performs the operation while viewing the area on a screen (at right). The technique involves the use of tools and cameras inserted through small openings.

Know the Risks »

All surgery carries an element of risk, and back surgery is no exception. For example, anesthetics sometimes cause serious side effects, such as postoperative infection, bleeding, and neurological problems, though these are rare. Deep vein thrombosis (DVT)—a blood clot in the legs, which is often associated with immobility and can move to the lungs—is also a risk, but can usually be avoided if a proper assessment of whether you are at risk is made before your operation. And sometimes, even though surgery appears to have gone well, it does not relieve a patient's pain or increase mobility—nobody is sure why this is.

The important thing is to ask questions about what risks are involved in your proposed operation, enquire about how experienced your surgeon is and what his or her success rates are, and make your decision accordingly.

Diskectomy In this procedure (also known as a "laminotomy" or "laminoforaminectomy,"), a small part of the bone that is impinging on nerve roots is removed under general anesthetic. When an endoscope is used to perform the operation, it may be known as a "microdiskectomy."

Laminectomy The laminae are two broad plates of bone running from each side of each spinal process (lumps that you can feel in your backbone, see page 14) to complete the vertebral arch. In conditions such as spinal stenosis (page 116) and spondylolisthesis (page 93), they start to pressurize the spinal cord or nerve roots. In a laminectomy, either one or both of the laminae are removed surgically to relieve this pressure. In a laminotomy, only the mid-section of one lamina is removed. If it is found to be necessary to remove a large amount of bone, spinal fusion (see right) may also be performed.

Foraminotomy When a facet joint, also called a Z-joint (page 14), degenerates as a result of age, disease, or injury, it can put pressure on a nerve root (page 82 and page 116) where it passes through the vertebral opening—the foramen. In a foraminotomy, a small amount of the bone that is causing the problem is shaved away, together with any bony outgrowths, in order to open up the foramen and reduce the pressure. A "foraminectomy" involves the removal of larger amounts of bone and with this procedure spinal fusion (see below) is usually necessary, too.

Spinal fusion This procedure is used to treat problems such as disk degeneration and spinal stenosis (page 116), scoliosis (page 54), and sometimes kyphosis (page 52).

The aim is to prevent any motion between two vertebrae by "welding" the vertebrae together, which, in theory, reduces the risk of pain. This is done by inserting a bone graft between the vertebrae. Depending on the individual and their condition, the vertebrae are likely to be pinned together by a mixture of screws, rods, and plates to keep them stable while new bone grows to make the fusion stable and permanent.

Spinal fusion is most suitable for people who are prepared to work hard at the physical therapy (page 178) needed for rehabilitation and for restoration of movement, which can take between six months and a year. While many patients—as many as a third, by some estimates—do not recover full movement, most experience a relief of symptoms and improved quality of life.

Total disk replacement (TDR) Although somewhat controversial, there have been several disk replacement systems devised and utilized over

For those who are judged to be suitable, some experts feel that TDR may be an alternative to spinal fusion. Following a TDR operation, an intensive course of physical therapy (page 178) to help restore motion is an essential part of the rehabilitation program.

If long-term studies validate the procedure, disk replacement surgery may become routine. It seems that TDR is at least as effective as spinal fusion for relief of pain and recovery of function.

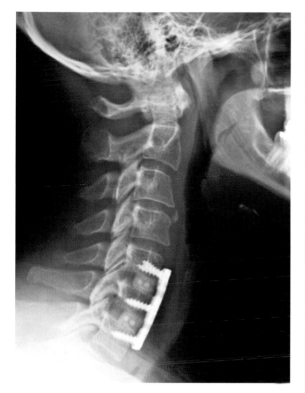

FUSION OF THE NECK VERTEBRAE
This X-ray shows metal braces in place following surgery to fuse the vertebrae. Bone grafts between the affected vetebrae are also visible.

the past few decades. European studies indicate that disk replacements succeed in about 70 to 80 percent of patients—but only if the surgeon is skillful and the patients are carefully selected. For example, people with osteoporosis (page 68) or other bone diseases, people who are obese, are smokers, have any form of malignancy or infection that affects the vertebrae, or have a variety of spinal defects, are not suitable candidates.

Watch for the Waves ▸▸

Radio waves have been used for many years as a treatment for back pain. At first, a technique called "radiofrequency" treatment was used to reduce the pain caused by nerve root problems. It killed off the nerves so that they could no longer relay pain signals to the brain. But this had obvious disadvantages because they could no longer transmit signals to the muscles. Then came "pulsed radiofrequency" treatment, which just "stunned" the nerves, but didn't kill them. Unfortunately, the treatment has to be repeated every two years or so to maintain effective pain relief.

A new treatment Magnetic resonance-guided ultrasound surgery, has been developed in which the facet joints and nerves are bombarded with waves of ultrasound. So far the technique has only been used on a few patients, but they reported a 62 percent reduction in pain and a 55 percent decrease in disability. Further trials are necessary before doctors figure out how useful this treatment will be.

Help Yourself!

For the majority of back problems that are not serious and clear up on their own within a week or two, self-help up front can play a part in reducing pain, hastening recovery, and preventing a recurrence. The exception is a serious injury. In this case the affected person should not be moved in any way; call 911 instead.

There are four mainstays to the self-help treatment of back problems: ice, medication, heat, and stretching exercises. Other self-help techniques include relaxation (page 162), massage therapy (page 186), and learning how to achieve and maintain good posture (page 148).

Always remember, if pain from an apparently minor problem lasts for longer than two weeks, is becoming worse, or if you suspect that there may be something more seriously wrong, do not rely on self-help, but consult your family physician.

Ice Place an ice pack on the site of any soft-tissue (muscle, ligament, or tendon) injury as soon as possible. Leave it there for no more than 20 minutes, then take it off for 20 minutes. Continue this on/off cycle for several hours. Applying ice has many virtues: it reduces inflammation, numbs sore tissues, slows pain signals to the brain, and reduces tissue damage. Never place ice on bare skin—you could could cause serious frost damage. If you do not have an ice pack, use a ice cubes or a pack of frozen peas wrapped in a washcloth or towel.

Medication Anti-inflammatory medications (NSAIDs, page 204), such as ibuprofen, and other painkillers, such as acetaminophen, are both useful and available over-the-counter. But make sure that you do not exceed the recommended dosage, and do not continue taking them for more than a few days before seeking medical advice. Remember, too, that all drugs have possible side effects and may interact with other medications. If you take other medications, check with your family physician before taking anything that hasn't been prescribed.

Heat After the first 24 hours, alternate ice on the site of the injury with heat; after 48 hours, just use heat. You can use an electric heating pad bought from a pharmacy, a hot-water bottle (use one with a cover or wrap it in a towel), or a self-sticking iron oxide thermal wrap. Heat increases the flow of blood, with its payload of oxygen and nutrients to the area. It also stimulates sensory nerve endings to reduce the number and intensity of pain signals sent to the brain. And it relaxes the muscles.

COOL IT
A store-bought ice pack is a convenient way of applying cold to an aching back.

Stretching exercises Start with general stretching exercises as you soon as you can, but do not push through any pain. Choose from the exercises described earlier in this book, whether for neck and shoulder injuries (page 96) or mid- and low-back problems (page 134). Perform your chosen exercises twice daily, and after you have recovered from your back problem, build them into your daily routine to help prevent any recurrence.

Braces Wearing a brace or support can sometimes provide comfort and a sense of security while you are recovering from a muscle or ligament strain. Some types may also help protect fractures while they are healing.

Most physical therapists advise against wearing a brace all the time—and not at all after the injury has healed. There is a risk of becoming psychologically reliant on it in that you may develop an unjustified fear of further injury if you don't wear one, and this may inhibit your full recovery. Ask your physician or physical therapist for advice on what type would be most suitable in your case. Here are some of the braces available:

- **Neck collar** A rigid neck support may increase neck stability in situations in which it might be at risk, such as when traveling. A soft neck collar does not provide effective support for an injured neck, but wearing one off and on for a few days following an injury or strain can be comforting.
- **Sacroiliac brace** This type of belt sits below the waist and provides a sense of support for those with low-back pain, buttock pain, or sacroiliac problems (page 124). A sacroiliac brace is particularly useful if you have to twist and turn as part of your daily routine—for example, when doing household chores.

- **Lower back brace** This is a belt that is designed to help your muscles support your lower back. This type of brace is especially useful if you have a problem affecting your lower back, but cannot avoid lifting and carrying.

Lumbar roll If you have a tendency to low-back pain, you can fit a lumbar roll to your chair. Lumbar rolls are also available for car seats, and some are even built in. They help maintain the natural lumbar curve, which is vital if you have a low-back problem.

Stay On Your Feet ▸▸

At one time, bed rest used to be advised as the first step to recovery for a back problem, but it is no longer thought to be effective. In fact, staying in bed for longer than 48 hours appears to prolong the problem, even in cases of severe pain. So stay on your feet and continue with your normal daily activities as far as possible.

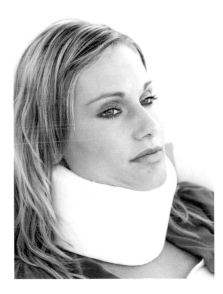

NECK SUPPORT
A soft neck collar can provide welcome comfort in the first couple of days after an injury. But don't use one for too long or you risk increased neck stiffness later on.

Resources

On these pages you'll find websites and contact details for organizations whose work and expertise may be relevant to your back problem. But your first port of call should be your family physician, who will know you and be aware of any existing medical problems—besides, there is nothing better than a person-to-person consultation. Use these sites to amplify what you are told about your diagnosis and treatment.

GENERAL

The American College of Physicians (ACP)
190 N Independence Mall West,
Philadelphia, PA 19106-1572
www.acponline.org
Phone: 800-523-1546, x2600; or
215-351-2600

The American Pain Society
4700 W. Lake Ave.,
Glenview, IL 60025
www.ampainsoc.org
Phone: 847-375-4715
Fax: 866-574-2654, 847-375-6479

INFORMATION WEBSITES

University of Maryland Spine Program
www.umm.edu/spinecenter

spine-health
www.spine-health.com

WebMD
www.webmd.com
www.webmd.com/back-pain/tc/back-problems-and-injuries-check-your-symptoms

The Mayo Clinic
www.mayoclinic.com

MedlinePlus
www.nlm.nih.gov/medlineplus/

TREATMENTS AND THERAPIES

Physical Therapy
The American Physical Therapy Association
1111 North Fairfax St.,
Alexandria, VA 22314-1488
www.apta.org
Phone: 800-999-2782
TDD: 703-683-6748
Fax: 703-684-7343

Osteopathic Medicine
The American Osteopathic Association (AOA-US)
1090 Vermont Ave., NW, Ste. 500
Washington, D.C. 20005
www.osteopathic.org
Phone: 800-962-9008
Local: 202-414-0140
Fax: (202) 544-3525

Chiropractic
The American Chiropractic Association
1701 Clarendon Blvd.,
Arlington, VA 22209
www.acatoday.org
Phone: 703-276-8800
Fax: 703-243-2593

Massage Therapy
National Certification Board for Therapeutic Massage and Bodywork (NCBTMB)
1901 South Meyers Rd., Suite 240,
Oakbrook Terrace, IL 60181
www.ncbtmb.org
Phone: 630-627-8000

The Alexander Technique
The American Society for the Alexander Technique (AmSAT)
PO Box 2307,
Dayton, OH 45401-2307
www.amsatonline.org
Phone: 800-473-0620 or 937-586-3732
Fax: 937-586-3699

The Pilates Method
The Pilates Method Alliance
PO Box 370906,
Miami, FL 33137-0906
www.pilatesmethodalliance.org
Phone: 866-573-4945
Local: 305-573-4946
Fax: 305-573-4461

Acupuncture
The American Academy of Medical Acupuncture (AAMA)
1970 E. Grand Ave., Suite 330,
El Segundo, California 90245
www.medicalacupuncture.org
Phone: 310-364-0193

Shiatsu
The American Organization for Bodywork Therapies of Asia (AOBTA)
1010 Haddonfield-Berlin Rd., Suite 408,
Voorhees, NJ 08043-3514
www.aobta.org
Phone: 856-782-1616
Fax: 856-782-1653

Surgery
The American Academy of Orthopaedic Surgeons (AAOS)
6300 North River Rd.,
Rosemont, IL 60018-4262
www.aaos.org
Phone: 847-823-7186
Fax: 847-823-8125

Medications
U.S. Food and Drug Administration (FDA)
10903 New Hampshire Ave.,
Silver Spring, MD 20993
www.fda.gov/drugs
Phone: 888-463-6332

Index

Acknowledgments

The author, Jenny Sutcliffe, would like to thank the following for their support and advice: Justin Elliot of the American Physical Therapy Association; Tom Perryman for advice on biomechanics and exercises. Special thanks are due to Nigel, with love, without whom the book would not have been written in such unusual circumstances.

Thanks are due to the American Academy of Orthopaedic Surgeons for permission to use the quotation on page 83.

Marshall Editions would like to thank the following agencies for supplying images for inclusion in this book:

2c Shutterstock/angelo gilardelli 6c Shutterstock/ Monkey Business Images 8tl Shutterstock/forestpath 9b Shutterstock/Christina Richards 11c Shutterstock/Yuri Arcurs 12c Shutterstock/Andresr 16bl Amanda Williams 16br Amanda Williams 17bl Amanda Williams 17br Shutterstock/ Guryanov Andrey Vladimirovich 19tr Amanda Williams 20bl Amanda Williams 22tr Shutterstock/meunierd 24b Barnaby Hewlett 26bl Shutterstock/Jiri Miklo 27tr Shutterstock/ auremar 28c Shutterstock/Flashon Studio 31c Shutterstock/ wavebreakmedia ltd 33tr Shutterstock/Kzenon 36bl Shutterstock/Yuri Arcurs 37r iStockphoto/Pali Rao 39br Shutterstock/StockLite 40b Shutterstock/Yuri Arcurs 42bl Shutterstock/Monkey Business Images 44tl Shutterstock/ luchschen 44tr Shutterstock/jannoon028 45tl Shutterstock/ Monkey Business Images 45tr Shutterstock/Christina Richards 46c Shutterstock/lev dolgachov 49c Shutterstock/ Yuri Arcurs 50bl Shutterstock/Monkey Business Images 51tr Shutterstock/Stanislav Komogorov 52tr iStockphoto/Red_ Frog 52bc iStockphoto/Red_Frog 54bl iStockphoto/Red_ Frog 56bl iStockphoto/Red_Frog 58cr Amanda Williams 59br Shutterstock/Kitch Bain 60bc Shutterstock/StockLite 61br Getty Images/Dorling Kindersley 62cr Amanda Williams 63tl Schermuly Design Co./Hugh Schermuly 63br Shutterstock/michaeljung 64bc Shutterstock/Juri 65cr Shutterstock/prism68 66tr iStockphoto/Red_Frog 68tr Science Photo Library/Susumu Nishinaga 68cr Getty Images/Alan Boyde 72c Shutterstock/T Anderson 75c Shutterstock/Diego Cervo 77tr Shutterstock/Diego Cervo 79b Shutterstock/IMAGENFX 81t Shutterstock/ prochasson frederic 83t Shutterstock/Alexander Raths 84c Shutterstock/Apple's Eyes Studio 85tr Shutterstock/Lisa F. Young 93c Shutterstock/Yuri Arcurs 95b Shutterstock/ Monkey Business Images 102c Shutterstock/grafvision 105c Shutterstock/Vasily Smirnov 106bl Shutterstock/ Randall Reed 106br Shutterstock/Randall Reed 107br Shutterstock/Zai Aragon 108l Shutterstock/Randall Reed 108tr Shutterstock/Randall Reed 109r Shutterstock/ stefanolunardi 111bc Shutterstock/Gorilla 114cl Shutterstock/ Dmitriy Shironosov 117tc Shutterstock/Adam Gregor 119tr

Shutterstock/iofoto 120bl Shutterstock/Randall Reed 121tc Shutterstock/Groomee 123br Shutterstock/Henrik Winther Andersen 125br Shutterstock/StockLite 126cr Shutterstock/ Monkey Business Images 127tr Shutterstock /Alexander Raths 128tr Shutterstock/marema 130bl Shutterstock/ PHB.cz (Richard Semik) 131tr Shutterstock/claires 131cr Shutterstock/claires 133br Getty Images/Kirk Mastin 142c Shutterstock/Yuri Arcurs 144c Shutterstock/Korionov 145tr Shutterstock/Kzenon 146bl Shutterstock/Warren Goldswain 147tr Shutterstock/Monkey Business Images 152cl Shutterstock/Marcin Balcerzak 154tr Shutterstock/ Kurhan 155cr Shutterstock/auremar 157br Shutterstock/ Martin Novak 158cr Shutterstock/wavebreakmedia ltd 161btl Shutterstock/Denis Pepin 161btr Shutterstock/Karen Struthers 161bbl Shutterstock/Morgan Lane Photography 161bbc Shutterstock/Tina Rencelj 161bbr Shutterstock/ Morgan Lane Photography 162tr Shutterstock/marema 172c Shutterstock/Juriah Mosin 175c Shutterstock/ NotarYES 176tr Shutterstock/Monkey Business Images 177tl Shutterstock/Yuri Arcurs 177tc Shutterstock/Borys Shevchuk 177tr Shutterstock/Konstantin Chagin 179tr Getty Images/Dougal Waters 181tl Shutterstock/Monkey Business Images 183bl Shutterstock/Monkey Business Images 185b Shutterstock/wavebreakmedia ltd 189c Getty Images/John Howard 190bl Science Photo Library/ Horacio Sormani 191br Shutterstock/Yuri Arcurs 192bl iStockphoto/kristian sekulic 197tc Shutterstock/iofoto 198cr Shutterstock/Monkey Business Images 201tr iStockphoto/ Aifos 203br Shutterstock/Rob Byron 204cr Shutterstock/ isak55 205bl Shutterstock/olly 209br Shutterstock/Martin Lízal 210tr Science Photo Library/Zephyr 211c Science Photo Library/Arno Massee 213tl Shutterstock/Anthony Ricci 214bl Shutterstock/liveostockimages 215br Shutterstock/ wavebreakmedia ltd

Illustrations on pages 16, 17, 19, 20, 58, 62 Amanda Williams

All step-by-step and other images are the copyright of Marshall Editions.

Schermuly Design Co would like to thank the following for their help in the preparation of this book: Lindsay Kaubi (for proofreading); Helen Snaith (for the index); and our models Daisy Brodskis, Chenade Laroy John, Andrew McGonigle, and Annameka Porter-Sinclair.

While every effort has been made to credit contributors, Marshall Editions would like to apologize should there have been any omissions or errors and would be pleased to make the appropriate correction to future editions of the book.